CANCER ETIOLOGY, DIAGNOSIS AND TREATMENTS

HEAD AND NECK CANCER

EPIDEMIOLOGY, MANAGEMENT AND TREATMENT OUTCOMES

Cancer Etiology, Diagnosis and Treatments

Additional books in this series can be found on Nova's website under the Series tab.

Additional e-books in this series can be found on Nova's website under the e-book tab.

CANCER ETIOLOGY, DIAGNOSIS AND TREATMENTS

HEAD AND NECK CANCER

EPIDEMIOLOGY, MANAGEMENT AND TREATMENT OUTCOMES

MADISON R. HALL

EDITOR

NOVA BIOMEDICAL

New York

NOTICE TO THE READER

Library of Congress Cataloging-in-Publication Data

ISBN: 978-1-63482-113-1

Library of Congress Control Number: 2015931170

Published by Nova Science Publishers, Inc. † New York

Contents

Preface

Over 50,000 new cases of head and neck cancer are diagnosed each year in the United States. The majority of these are squamous cell carcinoma (HNSCC), associated with human papillomavirus infection and carcinogenic behaviors such as tobacco use and alcohol consumption. Although these are more common, there are several other causes that this book addresses. This book examines the epidemiology of head and neck cancer. It discusses the management of head neck cancer as well as treatment outcomes.

Chapter 1 - Oral mucositis (OM) is among the most undesirable, painful, and expensive toxicities of cytotoxic cancer therapy; furthermore, it is disheartening for patients and frustrating for caregivers. Accurate assessment of the incidence of OM has been elusive, but accumulating data suggests that reported OM frequency is significantly less than its actual occurrence. It has been suggested that over 90% of head and neck cancer (HNC) patients receiving radiotherapy (RT) with concurrent cisplatin experience severe OM, with symptoms of extreme pain, mucosal ulceration and consequent limitations in swallowing and achieving adequate nutritional intake. This panoply of symptoms inevitably impacts patients' quality of life (QOL) and their willingness to continue treatment. In spite of all the advances made in understanding the pathophysiology of OM, there is still no prophylactic therapy with proven efficacy. Strategies to limit the extent of OM and to manage its symptomatology include basic oral care, supportive medications, nutritional support, and targeting aggressive treatments to high-risk patients. This review focuses on OM recognition, preventive measurements, and symptom-management strategies.

Chapter 2 - Over 50,000 new cases of head and neck cancer are diagnosed each year in the United States. The majority of these are squamous cell carcinoma (HNSCC), associated with human papillomavirus infection and carcinogenic behaviors such as tobacco use and alcohol consumption. Despite advances in both treatment and diagnostic technology, head and neck mortality rates have significantly decreased only for those cancers associated with positive HPV status. While early stage cancers can be effectively cured at a rate of up to 90%, there is still a subset comprising at least 10% of patients who experience recurrence and the associated devastation of repeated surgery, radiation, chemotherapy, and decreased survival despite appropriate and adequate treatment of the initial tumor. It is incumbent upon the medical community to further its understanding of the biology of HNSCC in order to delineate why and how some patients recur or persist while others remain disease free, and to develop effective methods to identify and address this treatment-resistant group. Recent head and neck research derived from both the leukemia and breast cancer fields have suggested that a small subset of progenitor cancer stem cells found in head and neck tumors may play a role in the disease progression of patients who experience disease persistence or recurrence. These studies have demonstrated that pluripotent, self-renewing cancer stem cells result in a hierarchical differentiation of epithelial tumors in the head and neck with reproduction of the original, heterogenous tumor phenotype in xenografts. Traditional thinking about oncogenesis endorses the theory of repeated cellular insult leading to multiple genetic mutations in the transformation of normal epithelial cells into tumor cells capable of unregulated reproduction and proliferation. There is growing evidence that the cancer stem cell theory should be considered in addition to this traditionally accepted stochastic model of tumorigenesis. This relatively new model of tumor development not only encourages a new way of thinking about the management of HNSCC, but suggests new molecular and genetic targets for chemotherapy and radiation therapy. Additionally, it may provide further rationale for multidrug resistant tumors, radio-resistant tumors, and late recurrence patterns, which are not explained by current stochastic models. This essay is a review of the current theories and findings in head and neck squamous cell cancer stem cell research, and a discussion of clinical implications of the findings to date.

Chapter 3 - Attenuation of the cell surface receptor (epidermal growth factor receptor, EGFR) mediated signaling cascade is a proven effective treatment approach in treating epithelial malignancies. The receptor tyrosine kinase (RTK) could be activated by a number of growth factors reversibly such as EGF, TGF-alpha, heregulins and HB-EGF. Inhibition of the activation of the EGFR receptor will block the activation of significant oncogenic signaling cascades including phosphatidylinositol-3-kinase (PI3K)/AKT pathway, mitogen-activated protein kinase (MAPK) pathway and JAK-STAT signaling pathway. Aberrations of the EGFR family are frequently observed in head and neck cancer. Specific genotypes will affect the treatment outcome and hence impact the prognosis of cancer patients. The use of EGFR tyrosine kinase inhibitors or specific antibodies is proven to be useful. However, the effects will gradually decline with the development of resistant phenotype. Recent data suggest that cancer cells will compensate the loss of EGFR-mediated signaling effects by increasing the signaling output of other EGFR members such as HER2. Human HER2 (ERBB2 or NEU) is one of the 4 members of the EGFR family. Gene amplification and protein overexpression of HER2 are found in head and neck cancer. Histological data revealed that protein overexpression of HER2 is site-specific with particular high frequency observed in a subset of cancers in head and neck regions. This chapter will provide a summary on HER2 with particular focus on the therapeutic aspects. Further, the significance of HER2 and the growing recognition of the particular functional roles in head and neck cancers will be addressed.

Chapter 4 - There is a general lack of public awareness on the daunting statistics of head and neck squamous cell carcinoma (HNSCC) when compared with other mainstay cancers such as breast and prostate cancers. HNSCC includes malignancies in five major anatomical sites, namely, oral cavity, oropharynx, nasopharynx, hypopharynx and larynx. HNSCC is diverse in nature both biologically and clinically. HNSCC is the 6th most common cancer globally with less than 50% survival beyond 5 years. Risk factors include smoking and alcohol consumption, betel nut chewing, wearing dentures, trauma to the gums and oral cavity as well as exposure to the human papillomavirus (HPV). HNSCC is more prevalent in men, however, the prevalence in women has been increasing due to changes in lifestyle over the last few decades. Whilst, smoking associated HNSCC is on the decline, HPV associated

HNSCC is increasing. The therapy of choice for newly diagnosed patients consists of combined modality treatment of surgery, chemotherapy and radiotherapy. Despite this aggressive first line treatment, over 30% of HNSCC patients develop locoregional and distant metastasis and succumb to the disease. Early diagnostics are the key to early interventions at the disease stage which can improve patient outcomes. This chapter aims to outline HNSCC trends and statistics, research based prognostic and diagnostic tools, treatments and patient management.

Chapter 5 - Head and neck squamous cell carcinoma (HNSCC), the sixth most common cancer in the world, is associated with risk factors such as the use of tobacco, alcohol, areca nut, and more recently apparent, chronic infection of human papillomavirus (HPV). HPV-positive HNSCC is associated with improved clinical outcomes despite presentation at more advanced stages. This article reviews the contribution of HPV to HNSCC development and tumorigenesis, and the current literature on HPV detection methods. It also discusses the role of microRNAs and epigenetic changes involved in HPV-positive tumours, its response to radiation therapy, and a discussion on prognosis.

Chapter 6 - The role of the Epstein-Barr virus (EBV), a ubiquitous lymphotropic human herpesvirus type 4, in the development of different tumours is not fully understood. In particular, it is unclear whether a specific strain or any strain of EBV circulating in the population is involved in carcinogenesis.

Elucidation of this problem for non-endemic regions, such as Russia, where EBV-associated tumours arise sporadically, is especially important. The present study aimed to study the status of EBV infection as well as the genetic structure of *LMP1* (a key oncogene of the virus) in patients with nasopharyngeal carcinoma (NPC) and in patients with other tumours of the oral cavity (OTOC). To this end, a comparative analysis of virus-specific antibody levels and the number of EBV DNA copies in the plasma of 22 NPC patients, 17 patients with OTOC and 19 blood donors (BDs) were tested. Special attention was paid to the investigation of polymorphisms of LMP1 in samples derived from tumour biopsies, blood lymphocytes and/or oropharyngeal lavages collected from the tested groups. The data reveal the presence of significantly higher anti-EBV antibody titres in the plasma of NPC compared to OTOC patients, but the number of DNA copies of the virus in the compared patient groups did not differ significantly. The analysis of the C-terminal region of the LMP1 sequences revealed that they closely matched LMP1 variants previously described by Edwards et al. (1999).

However, some characteristic features were also detected. In particular, the G212S substitution was not observed at all in the investigated LMP1 isolates. Overall, LMP1 variants from tumour samples of NPC and OTOC patients did not differ significantly either in the frequency of "highly oncogenic" LMP1 samples with 10 aa and/or 23 aa deletions ($LMP1^{China1}$ and/or $LMP1^{Med+}$), nor in the number of 11 aa repeats and the frequency of 5 aa motif insertions. No statistically significant differences were detected in the frequency of amino acid substitutions between LMP1 samples obtained from tumour biopsies and oropharyngeal lavages of both patient groups. Structurally similar LMP1 variants observed in both groups of patients are likely to reflect the polymorphism of EBV strains circulating in the general population. These data may indicate that, in both NPC and OTOC patients, EBV strains with similar LMP1 variants are found to persist. This observation allows us to suggest that, at least in non-endemic areas, EBV strains with any LMP1variants can induce NPC development, but the oncogenic potential of the virus in an infected individual may be realised only in the presence of additional exposure to harmful factors in the internal and external environment, such as chemical carcinogens, congenital or acquired immunodeficiency, a genetic predisposition to NPC development, and possibly dietary and other factors. To confirm the above assumption, a comprehensive and long-term study in several population groups with high and low levels of EBV-associated pathologies should be carried out.

Chapter 7 - The use of epidermal growth factor receptor (EGFR) inhibitors in several types of cancer has increased considerably in recent years. Currently they are approved in non-small cell lung cancer (NSCLC), pancreatic cancer, colorectal cancer (CRC) and squamous-cell carcinoma of the head and neck (SCCHN). Monoclonal antibodies against the EGFR (cetuximab, panitumumab) or EGFR tyrosine kinase inhibitors (gefitinib, erlotinib, lapatinib) are generally well tolerated and do not have the severe systemic side effect usually seen with cytotoxic drugs. A considerable number of patients treated with these EGFR inhibitors, however, develop dermatological side-effects, most frequently a papulopustular rash but also eczema, xerosis, telangiectasia, hyper-pigmentation, fissures, paronychia and hair changes. EGFR is normally expressed in the basal layer of the epidermis and contributes of the stimulation of epidermal growth, inhibition of differentiation and acceleration of wound healing. Inhibition of EGFR results in impaired growth, migration of keratinocytes, inflammatory chemokine expression of these cells and subsequent cutaneous injury. Desruption of these barrier may also promote bacterial overgrowth, further exarcebating injury to the cutaneous tissue.

Cetuximab related -skin toxicity have been reported in 60%-80% in patients with mCRC treated with cetuximab monotherapy with a similar frequency seen in trials of cetuximab in combination with chemotherapy. The most common adverse events among patients treated with cetuximab is the papulopustular rash. The onset of rash is early,generally developing over a period of six weeks after starting treatment. Incidencs and severity are usually dose dependent.

Effective and timing treatment of cetuximab related rash is mandatory to maximize the anti-tumor efficacy of cetuximab as well as maintaining the patients quality of life. Mild cases respond well to topical anti-infammatory therapy whereas tetracyclines and corticosteroids are needed to treat moderate to severe cases.

Available data suggests that the appearance and severity of skin rash is positively correlated with objective tumor response to cetuximab therapy and with overall survival. Data suggest that skin rash may serve as a surrogate marker of EGFR-targeted mAb efficacy. In patients receiving cetuximab monotherapy for refractory mCRC, longer survival times were observed in patients with rash of any grade as compared with patients experiencing no rash ($p = 0.02$).

In the BOND trial of cetuximab in combination with irinotecan as compared with cetuximab alone in patients with mCRC, response rates in patients with skin reaction were higher than rates in patients without skin reaction (25.8% vs. 6.3% in the combination group, 13.0% vs. 0% in the monotherapy group; $p = 0.005$).

Data from the CRYSTAL trial support this observation as the median PFS of patients without rash was 5,4 months compared to 9,4 months in patients with grade 2 and 11.3 in patients with grade 3 toxicity. The phase I/II of EVEREST study showed that response rate and skin toxicity both increased with dose escalation. The introduction of cetuximab in colorectal and head and neck cancer therapy had a significant impact on outcomes. A strategic approach to the management of skin toxicity will allow one to limit the incidence of skin rash, to improve patients` compliance and to optimize outcomes.

Chapter 8 - Laryngeal cancer is the second most common type of head and neck cancer worldwide. There exist many management options for laryngeal tumors today. Besides cure, organ preservation with retaining of function has been added as a primary goal of treatment. Numerous prognostic factors regarding patients undergoing treatment for laryngeal lesions have been evaluated in the literature.

Choice of treatment may be regarded as a major factor affecting prognosis. Multiple options are available for the management of laryngeal cancer. In the treatment of advanced cases, significant changes have been noted in recent years with a clear shift toward non-surgical, organ-preservation strategies.

As there appears to be worsening survival for laryngeal cancer, it has been proposed this may be related to the shift from surgery to chemoradiation.

For cases undergoing surgical treatment the prognostic significance of surgical margins cannot be overemphasized. It is common knowledge among surgeons that the aim of any tumor surgery with therapeutic intent should be histologically confirmed disease-free margins. It has been established that patients with laryngeal cancer exhibiting compromised margins have significantly higher rates of local recurrence and even show decreased survival. Status of surgical margins significantly affects oncologic outcome regardless of accompanying disease stage. Prognostic significance of tumor margins following laser resection shows more controversial outcomes.

Besides status of margins, N and T classification are widely considered to be significant prognostic factors. Comorbidity is an important factor affecting survival of patients with laryngeal malignancies. Age appears to be another prognostic factor although it has not proved to be independent. Same goes for the primary site of laryngeal cancer. Prognosis has traditionally been poorer for supraglottic carcinomas, compared to glottic lesions, due to the rich lymphatic drainage system and the relatively late appearance of symptoms. Histological grade of tumor has also been widely studied as a prognostic variable. Progression of dedifferentiation tends to worsen prognosis. The impact of tobacco use and alcohol consumption during treatment is still controversial. Studies have reported that long-term smoking is an independent factor of laryngeal cancer progression, and alcohol intake appears to have a well-known synergistic effect.

Lately, clinical trials have investigated the impact of viruses to prognostic outcome of laryngeal carcinomas. Accordingly, Human Papilloma virus status, specifically p16 strain, may be taken into account when considering organ preservation treatment for locally advanced larynngeal cancer. Patients with HPV/p16+ tumors have been shown to do favorably with chemoradiation, with improvement of disease specific survival (DSS) and local recurrence. Research for predictive value of biomarkers, and their impact on treatment decision making is still ongoing. Cyclin D1 expression in laryngeal cancer affects DSS and overall survival (OS).

Overexpression of EGFR is a poor prognostic factor, while low expression of BAK and NFκB were associated with good response in induction chemotherapy and chemoradiation respectively.

As many variables are considered significant in the management of laryngeal cancer, continuous evaluation may serve as a guide for more effective treatment strategies.

In: Head and Neck Cancer
Editor: Madison R. Hall

ISBN: 978-1-63482-113-1

Chapter 1

Management of Mucositis in Head and Neck Cancer Patients

***Marcelo Bonomi, MD,*[*] *and Katharine Batt, MD*[#]**
Medicine Section of Hematology and Medical Oncology
Wake Forest School of Medicine
Medical Center Boulevard, Winston-Salem, NC

Abstract

Oral mucositis (OM) is among the most undesirable, painful, and expensive toxicities of cytotoxic cancer therapy; furthermore, it is disheartening for patients and frustrating for caregivers. Accurate assessment of the incidence of OM has been elusive, but accumulating data suggests that reported OM frequency is significantly less than its actual occurrence. It has been suggested that over 90% of head and neck cancer (HNC) patients receiving radiotherapy (RT) with concurrent cisplatin experience severe OM, with symptoms of extreme pain, mucosal ulceration and consequent limitations in swallowing and achieving adequate nutritional intake. This panoply of symptoms inevitably impacts patients' quality of life (QOL) and their willingness to continue treatment. In spite of all the advances made in understanding the pathophysiology of OM, there is still no prophylactic therapy with proven efficacy. Strategies to limit the extent of OM and to manage its symptomatology include basic oral care, supportive medications, nutritional support, and targeting aggressive treatments to high-risk patients. This review focuses on OM recognition, preventive measurements, and symptom-management strategies.

Keywords: mucositis, head and neck cancer, chemotherapy and radiation, pain, nutrition

[*] Corresponding Author: e-mail: mbonomi@wakehealth.edu
[#] e-mail: kbatt@wakehealth.edu

Introduction

OM develops in the majority of patients receiving RT to the upper aero-digestive tract [1, 2], particularly those undergoing higher intensity radiation schedules (*ie* hyper-fractionated or accelerated RT [3, 4]) with concurrent cisplatin [5]. The prevalence of severe OM has been reported in 75-90% of this patient population [7]. With the addition of targeted therapies to current HNC anti-neoplastic treatment regimens, the risk of OM has increased. For example, cetuximab, when added to standard HNC chemo-radiation treatment (CRT) regimens, resulted in an increased prevalence of clinically significant mucositis when compared to CRT alone [6].

The relevance of OM extends from patient-related quality of life issues to provider-related concerns for timely treatment delivery and symptom minimization and finally, to broader health-system implications including resource utilization in treating OM. On the patient level, the literature reports severe OM is responsible for chemotherapy dose-reductions in two thirds of patients and complete discontinuation in a remaining one third of cases [8]. These complications can therefore, compromise the timely delivery of treatment, with resultant impact on local and distant recurrences. From the provider perspective, severe OM compromising the oropharynx, larynx, and hypopharynx, is extremely difficult to evaluate. Patients present with pain and dysphagia but the severity of inflammation, swallowing and mucosal compromise prevent direct assessment of the OM. The clinician is dependent therefore, on his/her best assessment based on patient symptom report. Given that 50% of patients can experience discomfort of the oropharynx and oral cavity for a prolonged period of time, even following resolution of visible OM [9], there are also long-term patient-related implications to OM [10, 11]. Finally, from a health system perspective, the incremental costs of treating HNC patients[1] with OM is >$17,000 per patient [12]. These costs are substantial and derive from hospitalization days, diagnostic tests, opioid use, and additional supportive measures, particularly an increased need for fluids and nutritional supplementation. Furthermore, the greater the severity of OM, the greater the associated costs of treatment.

Clinical Course and Impact of OM

The severity of OM ranges from superficial erythema with accompanying soreness, to full-thickness mucosal ulcerations and significant pain. These signs and symptoms are thought to correlate with the high levels of pro-inflammatory cytokines released during the development of OM [17, 18]. Among patients being treated for HNC, mucositis follows a predictable and well-documented course [13]. Of patients receiving myeloablative chemotherapy, RT, or both to the head and neck area, OM is the most commonly cited bothersome adverse event associated with the treatment. By the end of the first week of treatment with typical cumulative radiation doses of 10 Gy, patients evidence erythema of the oral mucosa and complain of a burning discomfort similar in intensity to a food burn. This relatively mild pain continues to escalate between the second and third week of treatment

[1] The economic evaluation accounted for both HNC patients as well as non-small cell lung cancer patients.

(with cumulative radiation doses of 20-30 Gy) as frank mucosal ulceration develops. Lesions at this stage often necessitate a modification in food intake and a marked increase in the need for analgesics. As radiation progresses, individual ulcers frequently coalesce, resulting in a confluent injury affecting many aspects of the oral mucosa. Pain intensifies and is often so severe that even with aggressive therapy, it can be very difficult to control [15]. With the abrupt appearance of severe, extensive ulcers and/or ulceration affecting the keratinized mucosa of the dorsal tongue, gingiva or hard palate, there is also an increased association with infection [13, 14].

It is clear then, that the clinical impact of OM is profound. Even when described as mild to moderate, OM is still associated with increased oral pain, weight loss, dietary modifications (including gastrostomy tube placement and subsequent use), dehydration, and reduced performance status [15]; even mild mucositis results in more frequent hospitalization and breaks in treatment [20]. Severe OM is associated with systemic findings of weight loss out of proportion to calorie intake, fatigue, anorexia, dehydration, and deconditioning. Ulcerations, in addition to causing severe pain, are also a frequent site of secondary infections. In myelosuppressed patients, an ulcerated area can act as a portal for systemic bacterial spread [16]. Severe OM therefore, is strongly associated with an increased risk of bacteremia and sepsis [19]. Finally, in patients who develop ulceration in high dose areas or in the posterior regions of the mucosa, symptoms may persist for several months beyond expected healing, causing ongoing symptomatology.

OM is therefore, associated with a wide range of symptoms as well as diminished quality of life (QOL) [7], significant health outcomes such as increased analgesic and antibiotic use, increased number of febrile days, prolonged lengths of hospitalization, needs for parenteral nutrition (and associated costs and infectious risks), and overall increased resource requirements and healthcare costs.

Assessment of Mucositis

It is critically important to develop and validate methods that can quantify the degree of OM experienced by patients in order to formulate appropriately targeted interventions. An emerging body of evidence suggests that assessments of OM should include a standardized instrument or combination of instruments measuring not only physical and functional factors, but patient-perceptions as well [18, 21]. The Multinational Association of Supportive Care in Cancer and the International Society for Oral Oncology (MASCC/ISOO) proposed that an OM assessment tool should be objective, sensitive, validated, reliable and easy to use in all clinical situations and applications. The World Health Organization (WHO) and the National Cancer Institute Common Terminology Criteria for Adverse Events (CTCAE) scales are the most commonly used yet neither tool assesses OM incorporating all the proposed criteria [8]. The WHO scale is easy to use but is based only on clinical observations of erythema and ulceration in combination with a patient's ability to maintain an oral diet [13]. The National Cancer Institute Common Terminology Criteria for Adverse Events (CTCAE) scale is frequently used in clinical trials to document the side effects caused by different anti-cancer therapies. Of note, the most recent version (v4.0) evaluates OM based on patient-reported variables such as pain, dysphagia and eating behavior in contrast to its predecessor (v3.0) that relied strictly on objective clinical findings such as erythema, ulceration and bleeding [22].

The v4.0, in line with more current thinking, better correlates with changes in QOL experienced while receiving CRT [23]. Available assessment tools still concentrate on clinician interpretation, despite evidence that patient-reported symptoms tend to be more severe than those recorded by physicians. As a consequence, the OM Daily Questionnaire (OMDQ) was created to record patient-reported OM outcomes on a daily basis without requiring clinic visits. This questionnaire, in addition to periodic clinical assessments, is designed to enable clinicians more rapid identification of OM and therefore, implement treatment and monitor subsequent improvements. In patients with laryngeal, oropharyngeal and/or hypopharyngeal cancers suffering from OM, direct visualization of the injured mucosa is extremely difficult, due to swelling, inflammation and pain preventing passage of a laryngoscope. Therefore, clinician and patient assessment exists as the only measure of treatment effectiveness [7].

Mucositis Prevention

A number of diverse interventions have been tested for the prevention of mucositis in HNC patients receiving CRT. Although many of these interventions (*i.e.* "magic mouthwash", chlorhexidine oral rinse) are available over the counter, used off-label or marketed as devices, the US Food and Drug Administration has approved none of these interventions for the prevention of OM. The Multinational Association of Supportive Care in Cancer and International Society of Oral Oncology (MASCC/ISOO) recently updated its clinical practice guidelines for mucositis prevention [24] to reflect the results of a systematic review reporting the beneficial effects of oral care protocols (combination of toothbrushing, flossing, and $\geq$ 1 mouth rinses to maintain oral hygiene) in the prevention of OM [24]. Although the data was not strong enough to support a full recommendation, there was enough positive evidence to favorably support the use of oral care protocols in preventing OM across all cancer treatment modalities. The same data also supported a suggestion *against* the use of chlorhexidine mouthwash for the prevention of OM in patients receiving RT for HNC [24].

Palifermin (keratinocyte growth factor-1) is the only agent approved by the US Food and Drug Administration and the European Medicines Agency for OM. This approval was based on a body of evidence that included a large, well-designed, randomized controlled trial as well as other supporting studies with recommendations for the use of palifermin for the prevention of OM in patients diagnosed with a hematologic malignancy planned to receive high-dose chemotherapy and total body irradiation followed by autologous stem cell transplantation [25]. In the HNC patient population, two double-blind, randomized, placebo-controlled trials assessed palifermin's efficacy in preventing OM [26, 27]. Both trials found that the physician-assessed benefit of palifermin was not paralleled in the patient-reported outcomes (PRO) (assessed through the mouth and throat soreness score). Adverse events reported by physicians were less accurate than those reported by PRO instruments. This has led to a suggestion that clinician-assessment tools be replaced by PROs. While there is likely general utility in a combined reported outcome [28], the resultant specific findings from these studies do not support the use of palifermin in preventing OM in HNC patients.

Another potential agent considered in the prevention of OM is that of the granulocyte-macrophage–colony-stimulating factor (GM-CSF). A review of the evidence not only suggests against the use of granulocyte-macrophage–colony-stimulating factor mouthwash, but it also finds reduced local tumor control when used during HNC RT. In a randomized, multicentric trial evaluating the preventive effect of granulocyte colony-stimulating factor (G-CSF) in patients receiving hyperfractionated RT or concomitant CRT, there was an unexpected increase in locoregional failures experienced by patients with stage III-IV squamous cell carcinoma of the head and neck area [29].

Benzydamine hydrochloride is a nonsteroidal anti-inflammatory drug that can inhibit the production of proinflammatory cytokines such as tumor necrosis factor-α and interleukin-1b. The MASCC/ISOO mucositis guidelines recommend the use of benzydamine mouthwash to prevent OM in patients with HNC who are receiving moderate-dose RT (up to 50 Gys) without concomitant chemotherapy. In the initial study, prophylactic use of benzydamine was assessed with patients undergoing a weekly clinical evaluation before, during and up to a maximum of 3 weeks following the completion of treatment. The benzydamine group demonstrated a 30% reduction in the incidence of erythema and radiation-induced ulcers. In addition, 33% of patients who received the study drug did not show any signs of radiation-induced ulceration as compared to 18% of patients who received placebo ($P = 0.037$). Patients receiving benzydamine rinses experienced a significant delay in the need for opioid analgesia as compared to the group on placebo drug ($P = < 0.05$). It is important to note however, that benzydamine did not show any clinical benefit in the group of patients that underwent a full course of accelerated RT [30]. In a second study evaluating the preventive effect of benzydamine oral rinses on the incidence of OM, subjects were again randomized to receive either the benzydamine rinses or a placebo drug. Unlike the previously described study, patients receiving a definitive course of RT or concomitant chemo-radiotherapy (CRT) for HNC were included in the study. Data from this study demonstrated that patients using the benzydamine rinses had only a 44% incidence of severe OM in comparison to the placebo group with a 79% incidence rate ($P = 0.001$) [31] of severe OM. In conclusion, both trials support the clinical utility in prophylactic use of benzydamine oral rinses with moderate doses of RT. Whether this conclusion can be broadened to patients receiving concomitant CRT is still unclear as the included sample size in both trials is too small from which to derive meaningful conclusions [30, 31].

Low-level laser therapy (LLLT) is a local application of a monochromatic, narrow-band, coherent light source. The MASCC/ISOO guidelines recommend LLLT for the prevention and treatment of OM in patients with tumors of the upper aero-digestive tract undergoing a full course of RT or CRT. The mechanism of action of LLLT remains unclear; it seems to have a protective effect at the cellular level during periods of oxidative stress in patients receiving head and neck RT [32]. In a recent metanalysis evaluating the preventive effect of LLLT, a reduction in the incidence of severe OM was observed. An even larger clinical benefit was detected when the analysis was restricted to trials that included patients who received LLLT doses greater than 1 Joule [33]. In a double-blind, randomized trial comparing two LLLT groups receiving daily LLLT of different dosages throughout the full course of RT[2], patients randomized to the high-dose LLLT (group 1) had less severe OM and reduced pain during RT [34]. It is important to note that there are inconsistencies in the reported clinical benefits of LLLT given the lack of standardized laser parameters and the differences in described dose levels reported in the literature.

[2] Group 1 LLLT dose: (60 nm/15 mW/3.8J/cm^2/spot size 4 mm^2; Group 2 LLLT dose: 660 nm/5 mW/1.3J/cm^2/spot size 4 mm^2.

Mucositis-Associated Pain

OM pain is reported in the majority of HNC patients undergoing treatment (8). It interferes with daily activities of living in approximately one-third of patients and with social activities and mood in 50 - 60% of patients (34). Pain usually arises from the activation of primary nociceptive afferents by tissue-damaging stimuli and the subsequent processing of this activity within the nociceptive system. It can also be generated within the nociceptive system either by a primary lesion or from overall dysfunction of the nervous system [35]. This type of pain is termed *neuropathic pain.* In a prospective study of patients with upper aero-digestive tract tumors, neuropathic pain was diagnosed in 56% of the studied subjects, although the primary pain presentation was a mixed picture [36].

As previously discussed, there is an increased frequency of patients with severe OM developing local infections, typically from Candida sp and Herpes virus family organisms [14, 37, 38]. Patients with local infections usually evidence higher pain and dysphagia complaints and often describe a "neuropathic" component during the pain episodes. The correlation between pain severity and infectious potential is important to recognize, as it implies not only the use of local anesthetic and analgesic medications, but appropriate antimycotics, antivirals and/or antibiotics. This subset of patients may evidence a pain severity that necessitates dose-escalating systemic analgesics in addition to local measures [37, 39].

Opioid Use for Management of Mucositis-Associated Pain

Morphine is the classic example of an opioid used for its analgesic effects. These effects result from its capacity to bind to opioid receptors in the central nervous system as well as those in the periphery. Basic science research suggests that morphine provides analgesic relief when locally applied to tissues damaged from a series of inflammatory events [40-42]; this has also been observed in clinical scenarios. In HNC pain, the topical use of morphine has further relevance. Firstly, morphine preferentially binds μ-receptors with local application [43]. Secondly, morphine has poor transmucosal and sublingual absorption. The absorption capacity of a given drug depends on the pK of the drug, the pH of the absorbing tissue and on the drug's lipid solubility [44-46]. Morphine is poorly lipid soluble and is optimally metabolized in a low pH. The oral cavity of a patient suffering from OM represents the ideal conditions for morphine with inflamed tissues creating direct receptor exposure in a low pH setting. In a study performed on HNC patients with primary tumors of the nasopharynx, oropharynx and oral cavity treated with concomitant CRT, twenty-six patients were randomized to morphine mouthwashes, or a formulation of "magic mouthwash", comprised of a mixture of magnesium aluminum hydroxide, viscous lidocaine and Benadryl. In the morphine arm, patients were instructed to use an oral rinse of 15 ml 2‰ morphine solution (2000 mg morphine diluted in 1000 ml of water) on an as needed basis every three hours, to avoid swallowing the oral rinses and to hold the mouthwash for 2 minutes. The "magic mouthwash" group was given the same instructions. In an analysis of the two groups, severe pain was experienced for, on average, 3.5 days less in the morphine group than in the group using "magic mouthwash". In addition, the majority of patients randomized to the "magic mouthwash" group also needed systemic opioids for pain control [47].

In another two-block pilot design study looking at patients with loco-regionally advanced upper aero-digestive tract tumors receiving definitive concomitant CRT, different morphine dosages and pK analyses of the solutions were performed. The patients were randomized to receive two differently dosed morphine oral rinses. Group 1 used 15 ml of 1‰ morphine solution; Group 2 used a 2‰ diluted morphine solution. In the extended phase (block 2), twenty-two patients were included to assess the efficacy and safety of the morphine solution diluted at 2‰. As expected, the group of patients receiving the higher dosed oral morphine solution (2‰) had better pain control than the group of patients receiving the lower dosed morphine solution (1‰). Interestingly, pK studies did not show any clinically significant differences between the two morphine concentrations [37].

Much of the evidence used to manage OM-associated pain is extrapolated from the bone marrow transplant literature. Another well-described systemic opioid with marked efficacy in this setting is fentanyl, a short-acting synthetic opioid with potent analgesic capabilities that can be administered intravenously or subcutaneously. The low molecular weight, high potency, and high lipid solubility of fentanyl allows it to be easily delivered transdermally via a 72-hour reservoir and controlled-release membrane with steady continual absorption through the skin into the microcirculation and ultimately, into the systemic bloodstream. Its available dosage strengths (12.5, 25, 50, 75, and 100 μgr/hr) allow easy titration of dosages, particularly in patients with compromised swallowing facilities.

Two prospective trials have shown that the routine use of transdermal fentanyl reduced the intensity of pain and improved the QOL of patients suffering from severe OM [48, 49]. In our experience, the transdermal use of fentanyl is the opioid of choice for HNC patients suffering from moderate to severe pain and compromised oral intake.

Adjuvant Analgesic Therapies

In patients with OM-associated neuropathic pain or a mixed pain picture, there is a definite role for adjuvant therapies [50]. In two retrospective studies evaluating the addition of gabapentin (median dosages of 2,700 mg/day) to OM-associated pain regimens in HNC patients treated with RT or concurrent CRT, there was decreased need for opioids to achieve good pain control [51, 52]. In a randomized trial evaluating opioids versus tricyclic antidepressants for OM-associated pain in HNC receiving RT, up to 40% of patients achieved sufficient pain control on tricyclic antidepressants alone [53]. Although no randomized trials to date have evaluated the use of anti-convulsivants and anti-depressants with opioids for the management of OM pain with neuropathic features, the available data supports their use in this clinical setting.

Doxepin hydrochloride is a tricyclic antidepressant that has demonstrated anesthetic and analgesic properties with topical administration. In a recent randomized trial organized by the Alliance Cooperative Group, oral rinses with Doxepin diminished the intensity of OM-associated pain as compared to placebo. However, no reduction in the opioid dosing was observed in this study [54]. This suggests that further studies are warranted to determine the role of doxepin oral rinses in the management of OM.

Nutrition, Hydration and Electrolyte Support during Treatment

In patients with malignancies of the upper aero-digestive tract, maintenance of adequate nutritional support is necessary to complete definitive CRT with curative intent. Without these supportive measures, the data has shown an increased risk of treatment interruptions, reducing the likelihood of tumor control and overall survival [55]. Regular dietary counseling during CRT appears to maintain and potentially, improve nutritional status [56]. Of particular importance is the achievement of protein-related goals as patients who maintain good protein stores have been shown to have less severe OM [57]. Recommendations for prophylactic enteral feeding as a means of maintaining adequate nutritional status include patients with a pre-treatment body mass index (BMI) less than 20, large primary tumors and/or with hypopharyngeal involvement, and/or with dysphagia prior to the start of treatment [58]. The duration of percutaneous endoscopic gastrostomy (PEG) tube feeding is considerably longer than that of naso-gastric tube (NGT) feeding [58, 59]. However, in a recent randomized trial evaluating the prophylactic use of PEG in patients with advanced HNC, prophylactic PEG use was associated with a significantly earlier start and longer use of enteral nutrition, fewer malnourished patients, and an improved health-related QOL at 6 months post-treatment. Of particular note, the group randomized to prophylactic PEG tube placement rated higher physical function, role function, and cognitive function as well as significantly less fatigue and feelings of illness [60]. There also appears to be a significant relationship between creatinine percent or BUN rise, and percent body weight loss in patients receiving concomitant CRT who do not have adequate nutritional support; dehydration associated with severe dysphagia during CRT and may be one of the causative factors [61]. In our experience, the routine addition of daily parenteral hydration during the last two weeks of radiotherapy is associated with improved renal function and less fatigue. The above data highlights the importance of routine nutritional counseling, the prophylactic use of PEG tubes, and hydration beyond that of standard hydration for patients with advanced HNC receiving CRT, particularly cisplatin.

Re-feeding syndrome is an under-recognized side effect of CRT treatments. It is usually defined as a potentially fatal syndrome, in which fluid and electrolyte shifts occur in malnourished patients who undergo artificial re-feeding by enteral or parenteral routes. It is a complex syndrome with hypophosphatemia as the hallmark feature. It can also feature changes in glucose, protein and fat metabolism, sodium and fluid balance abnormalities, thiamine deficiency, hypokalemia and hypomagnesaemia [62]. Patients with HNC have multiple risk factors for nutritional depletion such as malignancy-associated cachexia, dysphagia and odynophagia, iatrogenic treatment effects and pre-existing detrimental social behaviors and are therefore, at an increased risk of re-feeding syndrome. The main cause of re-feeding syndrome is rapid re-feeding following a period of undernourishment; the mode of feeding is not important. As a result of the metabolic changes in early starvation the body switches the main energy source from carbohydrate to protein and fat. The basal metabolic rate decreases by as much as 20–25%. As fasting continues, the body aims to conserve muscle and protein. Therefore, in an attempt to conserve ketone bodies, tissues switch to fatty acids for their energy source. An increase in blood levels of ketone bodies ensues, thereby stimulating the brain to convert to using ketone bodies as its main energy source. As a result, the liver decreases its rate of gluconeogenesis, thereby conserving muscle protein. As a result of all of these metabolic changes, several intracellular minerals become severely depleted, even though the serum concentrations of these minerals (including phosphate) may remain normal or near normal. When feeding is restarted, the body metabolism suddenly changes from catabolism to anabolism. The re-introduction of carbohydrates stimulates insulin release, leading to the uptake of glucose, potassium, magnesium phosphorus, and water into cells. Protein and fat synthesis are stimulated, further consuming minerals. As cells continue to be produced, available mineral reserves are consumed. These changes result in intra- and extracellular mineral deficits, leading to the clinical complications of re-feeding syndrome [60]. The importance of this problem was demonstrated in a survey of HNC patients receiving RT or CRT in which approximately 14% of patients were admitted with severe malnutrition and risk of re-feeding syndrome [63].

For effective prevention of re-feeding syndrome, a thorough nutritional assessment should be carried out before re-feeding is initiated. Important factors to assess include weight loss over time, current nutrition, existing social issues such as alcohol intake, and any underlying psychological issues. Baseline plasma electrolytes, especially phosphate, sodium, potassium, magnesium and glucose should be measured before feeding and closely monitored and corrected during feeding. For patients at high risk of developing re-feeding syndrome, repletion of calories should be started slowly (maximum 10 kcal/kg/24 h). This should be customized to individual patients' needs, and should increase slowly to meet needs over 4–7 days. In patients who are very malnourished (e.g. BMI less than 14 kg/m2 or negligible intake for 2 weeks or more), it has been recommended by NICE[3] guidelines that re-feeding should start at a maximum of 5 kcal/kg/24 h and take place with concomitant cardiac monitoring, due to the risk for arrhythmias [64]. In general, re-feeding should be introduced at no more than 50% of caloric requirements in patients who have eaten little or nothing for more than 5 days. The rate should then be increased if no re-feeding complications are detected on clinical and biochemical monitoring [64].

Oral, enteral or intravenous supplements of the following electrolytes should be given unless pre-feeding blood levels are high: potassium (usually 2–4 mmol/kg/day), phosphate (usually 0.3–0.6 mmol/kg/day) and magnesium (usually 0.2 mmol/kg/day intravenous, or 0.4 mmol/kg/day oral). Continuous assessment and correction of electrolyte imbalances should occur during re-feeding. Vitamin supplementation needs to be started immediately before and continued during the first 10 days of supplementation. The vitamins of particular concern include: oral thiamine 200–300 mg daily, vitamin B complex 1-2 tablets, three times daily (or full dose daily intravenous vitamin B preparation, if necessary) and a balanced multivitamin/trace element supplement once daily [64]. In conclusion, re-feeding syndrome is easy to prevent and detect, but often overlooked in HNC patients.

Conclusion and Future Directions

As our understanding of the pathophysiology of OM expands to include underlying molecular mechanisms, new potential targets for therapeutic interventions are being identified. To date, different topical and systemic medications have been used, yet no single

[3] NICE (National Institute for Health and Care Excellence) is an independent organization, established by the United Kingdom government, tasked to create guidelines regarding the appropriateness of drugs and treatments provided on the National Health System (NHS).

efficacious intervention or prophylactic agent has emerged as the leading treatment in the management of CRT-induced OM. Although several ongoing clinical trials are looking into manipulating the inflammatory cascade associated with CRT-induced tissue damage as point of intervention, standard preventive techniques are still primarly focused on adquate oral hygiene, pain management with topical and systemic analgesics and timely identification of symptomatic complaints that herald an infectious process. Supportive measures that address nutritional intake, electrolyte management, dehydration and aggressive pain management are still the best means of preventing OM.

References

[1] Trotti A, Bellm LA, Epstein JB, et al: Mucositis incidence, severity and associated outcomes in patients with head and neck cancer receiving radiotherapy with or without chemotherapy: a systematic literature review. *Radiother Oncol.* 66:253-62, 2003.

[2] Bourhis J, Lapeyre M, Tortochaux J, et al: Accelerated radiotherapy and concomitant high dose chemotherapy in non resectable stage IV locally advanced HNSCC: results of a GORTEC randomized trial. *Radiother Oncol.* 100:56-61, 2011.

[3] Awwad HK, Lotayef M, Shouman T, et al: Accelerated hyperfractionation (AHF) compared to conventional fractionation (CF) in the postoperative radiotherapy of locally advanced head and neck cancer: influence of proliferation. *Br. J. Cancer* 86:517-23, 2002.

[4] Vissink A, Jansma J, Spijkervet FK, et al: Oral sequelae of head and neck radiotherapy. *Crit. Rev. Oral Biol. Med.* 14:199-212, 2003.

[5] Traynor AM, Richards GM, Hartig GK, et al: Comprehensive IMRT plus weekly cisplatin for advanced head and neck cancer: the University of Wisconsin experience. *Head Neck* 32:599-606, 2010.

[6] Ang KK, Zhang Q, Rosenthal DI, et al: Randomized phase III trial of concurrent accelerated radiation plus cisplatin with or without cetuximab for stage III to IV head and neck carcinoma: RTOG 0522. *J. Clin. Oncol* 32:2940-50, 2014.

[7] Elting LS, Keefe DM, Sonis ST, et al: Patient-reported measurements of oral mucositis in head and neck cancer patients treated with radiotherapy with or without chemotherapy: demonstration of increased frequency, severity, resistance to palliation, and impact on quality of life. *Cancer* 113:2704-13, 2008.

[8] Sonis ST, Elting LS, Keefe D, et al: Perspectives on cancer therapy-induced mucosal injury: pathogenesis, measurement, epidemiology, and consequences for patients. *Cancer* 100:1995-2025, 2004.

[9] Epstein JB, Stewart KH: Radiation therapy and pain in patients with head and neck cancer. *Eur. J. Cancer B Oral. Oncol.* 29b:191-9, 1993.

[10] Raber-Durlacher JE, Elad S, Barasch A: Oral Mucositis. *Oral. Oncol.* 46:452-6, 2010.

[11] Rosenthal DI, Trotti A: Strategies for managing radiation-induced mucositis in head and neck cancer. *Semin Radiat Oncol* 19:29-34, 2009.

[12] Nonzee NJ, Dandade NA, Patel U, et al: Evaluating the supportive care costs of severe radiochemotherapy-induced mucositis and pharyngitis : results from a Northwestern University Costs of Cancer Program pilot study with head and neck and nonsmall cell

lung cancer patients who received care at a county hospital, a Veterans Administration hospital, or a comprehensive cancer care center. *Cancer* 113:1446-52, 2008.

[13] Sonis ST: Oral Mucositis. *Anticancer Drugs* 22:607-12, 2011.

[14] Nicolatou-Galitis O, Athanassiadou P, Kouloulias V, et al: Herpes simplex virus-1 (HSV-1) infection in radiation-induced oral mucositis. *Support Care Cancer* 14:753-62, 2006.

[15] Elting LS, Cooksley CD, Chambers MS, et al: Risk, outcomes, and costs of radiation-induced oral mucositis among patients with head-and-neck malignancies. *Int. J. Radiat Oncol Biol. Phys* 68:1110-20, 2007.

[16] Bodey GP, Rodriguez V, Chang HY, et al: Fever and infection in leukemic patients: a study of 494 consecutive patients. *Cancer* 41:1610-22, 1978.

[17] Haddad R, Sonis S, Posner M, et al: Randomized phase 2 study of concomitant chemoradiotherapy using weekly carboplatin/paclitaxel with or without daily subcutaneous amifostine in patients with locally advanced head and neck cancer. *Cancer* 115:4514-23, 2009.

[18] Murphy BA, Gilbert J, Ridner SH: Systemic and global toxicities of head and neck treatment. *Expert Rev. Anticancer Ther* 7:1043-53, 2007.

[19] Ruescher TJ, Sodeifi A, Scrivani SJ, et al: The impact of mucositis on alpha-hemolytic streptococcal infection in patients undergoing autologous bone marrow transplantation for hematologic malignancies. *Cancer* 82:2275-81, 1998.

[20] Vera-Llonch M, Oster G, Hagiwara M, et al: Oral mucositis in patients undergoing radiation treatment for head and neck carcinoma. *Cancer* 106:329-36, 2006.

[21] Sonis ST: Mucositis: The impact, biology and therapeutic opportunities of oral mucositis. *Oral Oncol* 45:1015-20, 2009.

[22] Institute NC: Common Terminology Criteria for Adverse Events v.3.0 and v.4.0 (CTCAE). Available at: http://ctep.cancer.gov.protocol Development/electronic _applications/ctc.htm, 2011.

[23] Liu YJ, Zhu GP, Guan XY: Comparison of the NCI-CTCAE version 4.0 and version 3.0 in assessing chemoradiation-induced oral mucositis for locally advanced nasopharyngeal carcinoma. *Oral Oncol* 48:554-9, 2012.

[24] Bensadoun RJ, Schubert MM, Lalla RV, et al: Amifostine in the management of radiation-induced and chemo-induced mucositis. *Support Care Cancer* 14:566-72, 2006.

[25] Spielberger R, Stiff P, Bensinger W, et al: Palifermin for oral mucositis after intensive therapy for hematologic cancers. *N. Engl. J. Med.* 351:2590-8, 2004.

[26] Henke M, Alfonsi M, Foa P, et al: Palifermin decreases severe oral mucositis of patients undergoing postoperative radiochemotherapy for head and neck cancer: a randomized, placebo-controlled trial. *J. Clin. Oncol.* 29:2815-20, 2011.

[27] Le QT, Kim HE, Schneider CJ, et al: Palifermin reduces severe mucositis in definitive chemoradiotherapy of locally advanced head and neck cancer: a randomized, placebo-controlled study. *J. Clin. Oncol* 29:2808-14, 2011.

[28] Basch E, Bennett A, Pietanza MC: Use of patient-reported outcomes to improve the predictive accuracy of clinician-reported adverse events. *J. Natl Cancer Inst* 103:1808-10, 2011.

[29] Staar S, Rudat V, Stuetzer H, et al: Intensified hyperfractionated accelerated radiotherapy limits the additional benefit of simultaneous chemotherapy--results of a

multicentric randomized German trial in advanced head-and-neck cancer. *Int. J. Radiat Oncol. Biol. Phys.* 50:1161-71, 2001.

[30] Epstein JB, Silverman S, Jr., Paggiarino DA, et al: Benzydamine HCl for prophylaxis of radiation-induced oral mucositis: results from a multicenter, randomized, double-blind, placebo-controlled clinical trial. *Cancer* 92:875-85, 2001.

[31] Kazemian A, Kamian S, Aghili M, et al: Benzydamine for prophylaxis of radiation-induced oral mucositis in head and neck cancers: a double-blind placebo-controlled randomized clinical trial. *Eur. J. Cancer Care* (Engl) 18:174-8, 2009.

[32] Bjordal JM, Bensadoun RJ, Tuner J, et al: A systematic review with meta-analysis of the effect of low-level laser therapy (LLLT) in cancer therapy-induced oral mucositis. *Support Care Cancer* 19:1069-77, 2011.

[33] Epstein JB, Elad S, Eliav E, et al: Orofacial pain in cancer: part II--clinical perspectives and management. *J. Dent Res* 86:506-18, 2007.

[34] Carvalho PA, Jaguar GC, Pellizzon AC, et al: Evaluation of low-level laser therapy in the prevention and treatment of radiation-induced mucositis: a double-blind randomized study in head and neck cancer patients. *Oral Oncol* 47:1176-81, 2011.

[35] Treede RD, Jensen TS, Campbell JN, et al: Neuropathic pain: redefinition and a grading system for clinical and research purposes. *Neurology* 70:1630-5, 2008.

[36] Potter J, Higginson IJ, Scadding JW, et al: Identifying neuropathic pain in patients with head and neck cancer: use of the Leeds Assessment of Neuropathic Symptoms and Signs Scale. *J. R. So.c Med.* 96:379-83, 2003.

[37] Cerchietti LC, Navigante AH, Korte MW, et al: Potential utility of the peripheral analgesic properties of morphine in stomatitis-related pain: a pilot study. *Pain* 105:265-73, 2003.

[38] Deng Z, Kiyuna A, Hasegawa M, et al: Oral candidiasis in patients receiving radiation therapy for head and neck cancer. *Otolaryngol Head Neck Surg*. 143:242-7, 2010.

[39] LeBon B, Zeppetella G, Higginson IJ: Effectiveness of topical administration of opioids in palliative care: a systematic review. *J. Pain Symptom Manage* 37:913-7, 2009.

[40] Hassan AH, Ableitner A, Stein C, et al: Inflammation of the rat paw enhances axonal transport of opioid receptors in the sciatic nerve and increases their density in the inflamed tissue. *Neuroscience* 55:185-95, 1993.

[41] Schafer M, Imai Y, Uhl GR, et al: Inflammation enhances peripheral mu-opioid receptor-mediated analgesia, but not mu-opioid receptor transcription in dorsal root ganglia. *Eur. J. Pharmacol.* 279:165-9, 1995.

[42] Likar R, Koppert W, Blatnig H, et al: Efficacy of peripheral morphine analgesia in inflamed, non-inflamed and perineural tissue of dental surgery patients. *J. Pain Symptom Manage* 21:330-7, 2001.

[43] Stein C: Peripheral mechanisms of opioid analgesia. *Anesth Analg* 76:182-91, 1993.

[44] Kaufman JJ, Semo NM, Koski WS: Microelectrometric titration measurement of the pKa's and partition and drug distribution coefficients of narcotics and narcotic antagonists and their pH and temperature dependence. *J. Med. Chem.* 18:647-55, 1975.

[45] Weinberg DS, Inturrisi CE, Reidenberg B, et al: Sublingual absorption of selected opioid analgesics. *Clin. Pharmacol Ther* 44:335-42, 1988.

[46] Ripamonti C, Bruera E: Rectal, buccal, and sublingual narcotics for the management of cancer pain. *J. Palliat Care* 7:30-5, 1991.

[47] Cerchietti LC, Navigante AH, Bonomi MR, et al: Effect of topical morphine for mucositis-associated pain following concomitant chemoradiotherapy for head and neck carcinoma. *Cancer* 95:2230-6, 2002.

[48] Kim JG, Sohn SK, Kim DH, et al: Effectiveness of transdermal fentanyl patch for treatment of acute pain due to oral mucositis in patients receiving stem cell transplantation. *Transplant Proc* 37:4488-91, 2005.

[49] Demarosi F, Lodi G, Soligo D, et al: Transdermal fentanyl in HSCT patients: an open trial using transdermal fentanyl for the treatment of oral mucositis pain. *Bone Marrow Transplant* 33:1247-51, 2004.

[50] Ling IS, Larsson B: Individualized pharmacological treatment of oral mucositis pain in patients with head and neck cancer receiving radiotherapy. *Support Care Cancer* 19:1343-50, 2011.

[51] Bar Ad V, Weinstein G, Dutta PR, et al: Gabapentin for the treatment of pain related to radiation-induced mucositis in patients with head and neck tumors treated with intensity-modulated radiation therapy. *Head Neck* 32:173-7, 2010.

[52] Bar Ad V, Weinstein G, Dutta PR, et al: Gabapentin for the treatment of pain syndrome related to radiation-induced mucositis in patients with head and neck cancer treated with concurrent chemoradiotherapy. *Cancer* 116:4206-13, 2010.

[53] Ehrnrooth E, Grau C, Zachariae R, et al: Randomized trial of opioids versus tricyclic antidepressants for radiation-induced mucositis pain in head and neck cancer. *Acta Oncol* 40:745-50, 2001.

[54] Leenstra JL, Miller RC, Qin R, et al: Doxepin rinse versus placebo in the treatment of acute oral mucositis pain in patients receiving head and neck radiotherapy with or without chemotherapy: a phase III, randomized, double-blind trial (NCCTG-N09C6 [Alliance]). *J. Clin. Oncol* 32:1571-7, 2014.

[55] Al-Othman MO, Amdur RJ, Morris CG, et al: Does feeding tube placement predict for long-term swallowing disability after radiotherapy for head and neck cancer? *Head Neck* 25:741-7, 2003.

[56] Garg S, Yoo J, Winquist E: Nutritional support for head and neck cancer patients receiving radiotherapy: a systematic review. *Support Care Cancer* 18:667-77, 2010.

[57] Zahn KL, Wong G, Bedrick EJ, et al: Relationship of protein and calorie intake to the severity of oral mucositis in patients with head and neck cancer receiving radiation therapy. *Head Neck* 34:655-62, 2012.

[58] Mekhail TM, Adelstein DJ, Rybicki LA, et al: Enteral nutrition during the treatment of head and neck carcinoma: is a percutaneous endoscopic gastrostomy tube preferable to a nasogastric tube? *Cancer* 91:1785-90, 2001.

[59] Corry J, Poon W, McPhee N, et al: Randomized study of percutaneous endoscopic gastrostomy versus nasogastric tubes for enteral feeding in head and neck cancer patients treated with (chemo)radiation. *J. Med. Imaging Radiat Oncol* 52:503-10, 2008.

[60] Ahmed S, Travis J, Mehanna H: Re-feeding syndrome in head and neck--prevention and management. *Oral Oncol* 47:792-6, 2011.

[61] Lin A, Jabbari S, Worden FP, et al: Metabolic abnormalities associated with weight loss during chemoirradiation of head-and-neck cancer. *Int. J. Radiat. Oncol Biol Phys.* 63:1413-8, 2005.

[62] Crook MA, Hally V, Panteli JV: The importance of the refeeding syndrome. *Nutrition* 17:632-7, 2001.

[63] Sheth CH, Sharp S, Walters ER: Enteral feeding in head and neck cancer patients at a UK cancer centre. *J. Hum. Nutr. Diet* 26:421-8, 2013.

[64] Guidelines N: Nutrition support in adults. http://www.nice.org.uk/page. aspx?o=cg032 accessed on 29/04/06 at 20:02, in Guidelines N (ed).

In: Head and Neck Cancer
Editor: Madison R. Hall

ISBN: 978-1-63482-113-1

Chapter 2

Cancer Stem Cell Theory in Head and Neck Squamous Cell Carcinoma: A Review of the Literature and Discussion of Clinical Implications

Christina Mimikos, DO and Vishal Gupt,a MD*
Roswell Park Cancer Institute, Buffalo, NY, US

Abstract

Over 50,000 new cases of head and neck cancer are diagnosed each year in the United States [1]. The majority of these are squamous cell carcinoma (HNSCC), associated with human papillomavirus infection and carcinogenic behaviors such as tobacco use and alcohol consumption. Despite advances in both treatment and diagnostic technology, head and neck mortality rates have significantly decreased only for those cancers associated with positive HPV status. While early stage cancers can be effectively cured at a rate of up to 90%, there is still a subset comprising at least 10% of patients who experience recurrence and the associated devastation of repeated surgery, radiation, chemotherapy, and decreased survival despite appropriate and adequate treatment of the initial tumor [2]. It is incumbent upon the medical community to further its understanding of the biology of HNSCC in order to delineate why and how some patients recur or persist while others remain disease free, and to develop effective methods to identify and address this treatment-resistant group. Recent head and neck research derived from both the leukemia and breast cancer fields have suggested that a small subset of progenitor cancer stem cells found in head and neck tumors may play a role in the disease progression of patients who experience disease persistence or recurrence. These studies have demonstrated that pluripotent, self-renewing cancer stem cells result in a hierarchical differentiation of epithelial tumors in the head and neck with reproduction of the original, heterogenous tumor phenotype in xenografts [3]. Traditional thinking about oncogenesis endorses the theory of repeated cellular insult leading to multiple genetic mutations in the transformation of normal epithelial cells into tumor cells capable of

* Coressponding Author: Vishal Gupta, MD (Vishal.Gupta@RoswellPark.Org)

unregulated reproduction and proliferation. There is growing evidence that the cancer stem cell theory should be considered in addition to this traditionally accepted stochastic model of tumorigenesis. This relatively new model of tumor development not only encourages a new way of thinking about the management of HNSCC, but suggests new molecular and genetic targets for chemotherapy and radiation therapy. Additionally, it may provide further rationale for multidrug resistant tumors, radio-resistant tumors, and late recurrence patterns, which are not explained by current stochastic models. This essay is a review of the current theories and findings in head and neck squamous cell cancer stem cell research, and a discussion of clinical implications of the findings to date.

Introduction

There is a wide spectrum of phenotypic variability between normal tissues and malignant neoplasms. Between these two extremes lies a continuum of progressive hyperplasia, metaplasia, dysplasia, and progressively less differentiated cellular phenotypes. In theory, a tumor mass descends from a single cell which undergoes unregulated clonal expansion, leading to the expectation that tumor specimens are composed of cells with a single genotype. In reality, tumor masses are composed of heterogeneous cells, with multiple genotypes and varying phenotypes and degrees of differentiation throughout the tumor bulk. There are several theories underlying this finding. One intuitive explanation in head and neck malignancies is that the effect of carcinogens is felt throughout the entirety of the mucosa, and that several cells at any given time may transform from normal to neoplastic. Thus, as many cells as were originally transformed would proliferate in a monoclonal fashion, producing a heterogeneous tumor bulk. Another possibility is the continued exposure of the newly proliferative, monoclonal mass to carcinogenic insult, resulting in continued random changes to the genome, thus spawning multiple generations of newly oncogenic clones with ever- increasing genomic instability. These theories of tumorigenesis are predisposed on the idea that all tumor cells are created equal, and that any one of the cells in a tumor mass is capable of spawning its own army of clones. Over the last twenty years, there has been an increasing body of evidence that all tumor cells are not created equal, and that only a very few cells within any given tumor have the potential to drive tumorigenesis, invasion, and metastasis [4].

Tumorigenesis

The prevailing dogma regarding carcinogenesis is that unregulated proliferation and dedifferentiation are the result of cumulative damage to DNA. The number of cellular insults required to permanently deregulate cellular growth is not universally agreed upon, however it has been accepted for decades that multiple genomic insults are required over time in order to escape the regulatory machinery of the cell cycle. The inactivation of tumor-suppressor genes, or the activation of proto-oncogenes is the result of these repeated insults. This is followed by the evolution of a malignant phenotype, an accumulation of the net events that precede it. This evolutionary continuum is well demonstrated in HNSCC, by the observable spectrum of premalignant lesions giving way to progressively higher-grade dysplasia, followed by in situ and finally invasive carcinoma.

Various models of tumorigenesis have been proposed to outline mechanisms by which tumors develop and grow. The stochastic (evolutionary) model proposes that every cancer cell has equal propensity to initiate and propagate tumors and metastases. This implies that phenotypic diversity in tumors is due to spontaneous shifts in cell phenotypes. This is supported in HNSCC by pre-neoplastic lesions which may extend beyond biopsy or surgical margins, in which local recurrences and secondary tumors appear [2].

In contrast, the hierarchical model describes a differentiation – like diversification from an initially monoclonal tumor cell lineage in which cells undergo asymmetrical division, producing copies of both themselves and more differentiated progenitor cells. This proposed pattern of asymmetrical division and differentiation of daughter cells is analogous to the renewal, growth, and differentiation undertaken by healthy epithelium without the oversight of the normal regulators of growth and division [5,6].

The question that naturally arises from a discussion of these two viewpoints is one of cellular potential. Are all the cells in a tumor mass immortalized, capable of escaping senescence and crisis? Is every cell in a tumor truly capable of spawning an unrestricted number of clones, metastasizing, and initiating new tumor?

With the advancement of cancer stem cell research, these questions are now being answered. It appears that there is a hierarchy of tumorigenic potential, only made evident with the advent of technology such as fluorescence activated cell sorting (FACS), which allows the sorting of viable cells and examination of their behavior both in vitro and in xenograft models.

Stem Cell Theory

The stem cell hypothesis is derived from our understanding of stem cell concepts derived from embryogenesis, applied to the process of tumorigenesis [6]. Stem cell theory posits that tumors are not insular masses of proliferating cells, but rather can be viewed as "organs", complex tissues composed of transformed cells that interact with stromal cells within the tumor microenvironment [7]. It states that tumors are essentially composed of cells in three various states. The first are cancer stem cells (CSCs), the multi-potent, self-renewing, tumor-initiating cells which are capable of undergoing asymmetric cell division. These cells are largely quiescent, dividing only rarely to produce one daughter stem cell and one daughter transit-amplifying cell. Transit-amplifying (progenitor) cells compose the rapidly proliferating bulk of the tumor tissue and are capable of undergoing a large number of symmetric cell divisions before their descendants become fully differentiated. The third types of cells are post-mitotic differentiated cells, which will no longer undergo division. Neither transit-amplifying nor post-mitotic cells have the ability to initiate metastases or seed new tumors, as they are not self-renewing, despite their lack of normal cellular regulation by tumor suppressor genes [7]. This differentiation of tumor stem cells into tumorigenic and non-tumorigenic cells is supported by the work of Pierce and Wallace, who showed that tritiated thymidine labeled mouse squamous carcinoma cells were capable of generating non-tumorigenic keratinocytes [8]. Further, Schatton et al. demonstrated that tumor growth could be halted by selective killing of CSCs. CSCs themselves are relatively quiescent relative to the multiplying, non –multi-potent tumor bulk, which allows them to evade therapies which target rapidly dividing cells [9].

Since the work of Lapidot et al. in the early 1990s, the idea of cancer stem cells contributing to treatment failure and cancer recurrence has been gaining both support and credibility [10]. CSCs were first identified in hematopoetic malignancies [11,12], and the first in vivo model of stem cell self renewal was developed in the leukemia field. Distinct stages of hematopoetic cell development were identified by surface markers, namely the stem cell progenitors which were found to be CD34+/CD38-8 and CD90-9. These cells were capable of initiating acute myeloid leukemia in nonobese diabetic / SCID mice. These cells were isolated either by immunostaining or by FACS sorting based on Hoechst 33342 dye exclusion. Importantly, some of these markers are expressed in normal tissue stem cells as well, and others are conserved between epithelial tumor types. Isolation of these subpopulations has identified which subsets of cells able to undergo asymmetric cell division and which have a greatly increased ability to produce tumors in immunodeficient mouse models relative to the bulk of the tumor cell population.

Since this initial model was developed, stem cells have been identified in a wide variety of solid tumors as well, including breast, colon, CNS, prostate, and pancreatic malignancies. Sub- or side populations of cells in several types of solid tumors that have been identified include CD44+/CD24- cells in breast cancers and CD 133+ cells in CNS tumor. These subpopulations were able to initiate tumors in NOD/SCID mice from as few as one hundred cells, as opposed to lower rates of tumor generation from tens of thousands of cells with other markers [13].

Regardless of tumor type, CSCs require the following characteristics to be classified as tumorigenic stem cells: 1) Only a small fraction of the cancer cells within a tumor have tumorigenic potential; 2) The cancer stem cell sub-population can be separated from other cancer cells by distinctive cell markers; 3) Tumors resulting from CSCs contain the mixed tumorigenic and non-tumorigenic cells of the original tumor, demonstrating CSC multi-potency; and 4) The cancer stem cell population can be serially transplanted or passaged through multiple generations, indicating that it is a self-renewing population [14].

The initial landmark work in stem cell theory in HNSCC has come from the laboratory of Prince et al., who identified CD44+cells as the only cells capable of generating tumors in vivo through serial passages in an immunodeficient mouse model. They found that the CD44+ cells had a primitive morphology, co-stain with the basal cell marker cytokeratin 5/14, and demonstrate high levels of BMI1, previously found to participate in self renewal and tumorigenesis. The tumors produced by these cells demonstrated original tumor cell heterogeneity. In contrast, the CD44- cells more closely resembled differentiated squamous epithelium and expressed the differentiation marker involucrin. The tumors produced by implantation of CD44+ cells also reproduced the heterogeneity of the original tumors. When CD44 + and – cells were injected into NOD/SCID mice, 20 of 31 injections of CD44+ cells formed tumors, whereas only 1 of 40 injections of CD44- cells was able to produce a tumor. As few as 5x10^3 gave rise to new tumors, where up to 5x10^5 cells of CD44- cells failed to form tumors. These findings strongly supported the stem cell hypothesis [14, 15].

Cancer stem cells are implicated in the virulence of aggressively metastatic and invasive carcinomas. This is thought to be mediated by the process of epithelial-mesenchymal transition, or EMT. EMT is a part of normal embryonic morphogenesis and cell migration, by which epithelial cells detach from their surrounding cellular niche, convert from an epithelial to more mesenchymal phenotype, express matrix degrading enzymes, become increasingly mobile, and display a heightened resistance to apoptosis [6]. Malignant epithelial cells may undergo EMT and begin to co-express mesodermal and endodermal markers, and demonstrate pluripotency once again. EMT is part of normal development, but aberrant activation of this cellular programming can contribute to various pathology, including fibrosis and carcinoma. It is proposed that cells which undergo EMT in carcinogenesis are able to detach from their cellular niche and migrate either invasively within adjacent tissue, or to distant sites in the body, while maintaining a stem cell phenotype capable of generating new tumor. Additionally, once migrating mesenchymal cells reach their destination, they can undergo mesenchymal – epithelial transition (MET) and begin generating new epithelial tumor [16].

The final tenant of stem cell theory is the acknowledgement of the stem cell microenvironment, or niche, as necessary for stem cell survival [17,18]. The quiescent, self-renewable state of the cell is predicated on cellular and non-cellular signals. Fuchs et al. proposed that non-epithelial stromal cells, inflammatory cells, and vasculature are the key components of the niche [19]. Krishnamurthy et al. have demonstrated that the majority of stem cells are located close to blood vessels, dependent not only on nutrition and oxygen from the vasculature, but also on endothelial cell factors for promotion of their survival and self-renewal [18].

Origins

The origins of CSCs remain unclear, and it has not yet been determined if they are oncogenically transformed normal epithelial stem cells, or partially differentiated progenitor (transit amplifying) cells which have undergone oncogenic transformation or epithelial mesenchymal transiition, and therefore assumed a more stem cell like character. In the work of Prince et al., it was noted that CD44+ cells were present in the basal layer of well to moderately well differentiated tumors, and absent in the more differentiated outter layers. It is unclear whether this indicates that CSCs derive from the basally located normal tissue stem cells, or whether they simple establish a niche nearly the basement membrane [3].

Stem Cell Markers

Currently there is no universal cancer stem cell marker. Therefore, significant time and energy has been devoted to the investigation of different markers in various types of malignancy. In HNSCC there are several promising candidates.

CD44 is a member of the transmembrane glycoprotein receptors that bind to hyaluronan. It has been shown that the CD44-hyaluronan interaction induces signaling events which promote tumor cell proliferation, migration, invasion, angiogenesis, and metastasis. Further, the stemness genes Nanog, BMI1, Notch 1 and Oct4 were up-regulated in CD44 cells. These cells were resistant to multiple apoptotic agents, and spend a longer time in the G2 phase of the cell cycle, possibly allowing for efficient repair of DNA damage [20] These CSCs cells also co stain for Cytokeratin 5/14, a marker of normal squamous epththelial stem and progenitor cells. Of note, staining for CK5/14 and Involucrin, a differentiated keratinocyte marker, were mutually exclusive. [3]. As Albers et al. point out, however, high numbers of CD44 cells were required to induce tumor growth in Prince's mouse model. Variant isoforms of CD44 have been investigated in HNSCC, with Wang et al. reporting that their line expressed at least 4 isoforms (standard (s), v3, v6, and v10), and that the expression of the non-standard variants correlated with advanced T stage, metastasis, perineural invasion, and radiation failure [21]. This is in stark contrast to the work of Mack et al., who found that comparision of CD44s to CD44v6 did not distinguish between normal and malignant epithelium in the head and neck [22]. Together, these findings suggest that further refinement of CD44 as marker for CSCs in HNSCC may be needed.

Aldehyde dehydrogenase (ALDH) is another marker under investigation in HNSCC CSCs. It has recently been shown to be a marker for CSCs in other epithelial tumors, including breast, lung, hepatic, and colon cancer [3,16,23]. ALDH is an intracellular enzyme involved in converting retinol to retinoic acid [24]. Its expression is also involved in EMT, which both functions to help cells retain stemness and aid in dissemination of disease. This marker has been found to be enriched in CSCs of breast and brain [25]. Recently, Krishnamurthy et al. investigated the role of ALDH in HNSCC. They demonstrated that cells with high ALDH activity exhibit stem cell behavior in HNSCC; 1000 CD44+/ALDH+ tumor cells were implanted into 15 mice, with 13 resultant tumors. Implantations of 10,000 ALDH-/CD44- cells produced tumors only 2 times in 15 implantations. Clay et al. also investigated the tumorigenic behavior of ALDH+ cells, and found that as few as 500 cells were able to create tumors, unlike ALDH- cells [23].

CD133 has been implicated in tumors of the HN, CNS, colon, pancreas, lung and liver. Like CD44, it is a transmembrane glycoprotein, and may have a role in regulating plasma membrane topology [16].

CD24 is a cell adhesion molecule used as a CSC marker in breast and pancreatic cancer. When co-expressed with CD44, cells possessed stem cell characteristics and demonstrated higher in vivo invasiveness [26].

EpCAM, or ESA, is an epithelial cell adhesion protein involved in Wnt signaling. It can be co-expressed with CD44, leading to a proliferative cell with epithelial characteristics, as opposed to mesenchymal characteristics [26].

Many factors under investigation modulate epithelial mesenchymal transition. Snail is a transcriptional repressor which is upregulated in EMT and modulated by IL-1beta. It regulates COX-2 dependent E cadherin expression, which is involved in cell to cell adhesion and recognition. Twist is another factor found to promote EMT and regulates several genes involved in differentiation, adhesion and proliferation [16].

BMI1 functions as a transcriptional repressor of senescence-inducing genes, implicated in the self- renewal of stem cells [27]. Tabor et al. delineated a side population from an both a cell line and from fresh human tumors which demonstrated CSC behavior, effluxed Hoechst 33342 dye, and expressed BMI1 at a level 4 fold higher than non-SP cells [13].

Markers which function in the maintainance of the stem cell phenotype include Oct-4, SOX2, and Nanog. Oct-4 is a transcription factor expressed in pluripotent embryonic stem cells which plays a central role in embryonic development, and may function as a master switch during differentiation by regulating stem cell pluripotency. SOX2 and Nanog are transcription factors which partner with Oct-4 in maintaining a stem cell phenotype [28,29].

ATP binding cassette transporters (ABC) have been used to identify cells with increased longevity. They efflux various drugs, including DNA binding dye Hoechst 33342. These cells are able to transport cytotoxic drugs out of the cell before they are able to cause DNA damage that would be detrimental to a stem cell. Their ability to efflux drugs far outstrips that of the limited ability of a more differentiated cell with limited proliferative potential [30]. These transporters are well characterized in breast cancer, with Trock et al. reporting that an average of 41% of breast tumors expressed the transporter ABCB1, and that those patients were three times more likely to be chemoresistant than patients without ABCB1 [31). This has not directly correlated to findings in head and neck tumors, however. Tabor et al. observed only a 1.4 increase in the ABC protein ABCG2 in their side population study, and proposed that an as yet unidentified secondary multidrug transporter protein was likely at work, given that the overexpression of ABCG2 was less than expected [13].

The CSC as a Theraputic Target

Patients with distant metastases from a primary HNSCC have a dismal prognosis, with median survival rates of 6-10 months [16]. The cancer stem cell is an attractive target for cancer therapy; paradoxically they have been shown to demonstrate resistance to standard chemotherapy and radiation treatments, and experimental populations of CSCs have been shown to be enriched 2-3 fold by standard chemotherapy treatments. While the main tumor bulk may respond well to the initial treatment, the CSC may lie quiescent and slowly dividing, thus evading conventional therapy aimed at rapidly dividing cells. This may account for the presence of highly aggressive recurrences and metastases in HNSCC patients which is unresponsive to chemotherapy or radiation, despite good response of the primary tumor. Sabisz et al. propose that increased ABC transporters, changed functionality of cell cycle checkpoints, elongated cell doubling, enhanced cell survival signaling, and increased DNA repair capacity are the mechanisms underlying CSC treatment resistance .

It is generally accepted that the derangement of apoptotic control is central to the development of cancer. As many chemotherapeutic agents and radiation depend on apoptosis resulting from DNA damage as a mechanism of drug induced death, this loss of apoptotic regulation may be part of the mechanism of chemoresistance in the CSC. However, there has not been consistent nor conclusive evidence that p53 mutation or over expression of BCL-2 alone are predictive of chemosensitivity in solid tumors [31].

Since CSCs make up such a small percentage of the overall tumor volume, effective targeted treatment will likely not reduce the tumor burden, but will instead make the tumor unable to grow further or regenerate when the majority of the cells succumb to treatment. Current treatment targets include the CSC niche, cellular pumps, stemness factors, signaling pathways, and the EMT pathway [31].

Tumors induce new vasculature as part of their growth, and as we have discussed, the CSC niche appears to be largely perivascular. Despite the accelerated angiogenesis, rapidly growing tumors can quickly outstrip their blood supply and become hypoxic, leading to necrosis. Without sufficient blood supply and tissue oxygen, the tumor becomes increasingly radio-resistant, and will increase production of tumor cell survival factors like hypoxia inducing factor 1alpha, and vascular endothelial growth factor (VEGF) [31]. VEGF normally functions to increase vascular permeability and promote angiogenesis. VEGF is the target of bevacizumab, a monoclonal antibody. It is directly cytotoxic to endothelial cells, can target VEGF and its receptors, instead of needing to gain access to the tumor mass. In theory, this decreases the proportion of hypoxic cells, so that increased oxygen content may allow the production of reactive oxygen species, augmenting the effectiveness of radiotherapy. Caution should be exercised, however, as it has been demonstrated that anti-angiogenic therapy may accelerate malignant progression as tumor cells require an invasive phenotype in order to escape the suddenly unhospitable microenvironment [32, 33]. Krishnamurthy et al. also examined iCaspase-9, a caspase based artificial death switch to selectively eliminate tumor-associated blood vessels in xenografts. They were successful in reducing the fraction of CSC in xenograft models with this method [18]. Epidermal growth factor receptors (EGF-R) are another target of stem cell niche therapy. EGF drives cell growth, proliferation, and differentiation. Inhibition of its cell surface receptor deprives the cell of the proliferative and anti-apoptotic signals. EGFR expression is not specific to CSCs, but has been shown to be upregulated in ALDH+ clonal populations, and the inhibition of EGFR has been shown to reduce stem cell fractions in those populations [34].

EGFR inhibitors (gefitinib), Src/Abl kinase inhibitors (imatinib mesylate), and tyrosine kinase inhibitors have been investigated as a possible methods by which to inhibit ABC transporters MDR1/ABCB1, MRP1/ABCC1, and ABCG2/BCRP [35,36]. By halting the efflux of multiple chemotherapeutic agents, the drug resistance of the CSC may be able to be overcome. Other drugs such as calcium channel blockers, cyclosporine, tamoxifen, valspodar, and zosuquidar have been found to inhibit ABC pumps and decrease the clearance of chemotherapeutic agents [26]. Recently ALDH enzymes have been found to coordinate with ABC transporters, and inhibition of ALDH activity has been associated with increased sensitization of cell lines to radio and chemo therapy [37] .

Targeting stemness challenges that ability of a CSC to remain quiescent. Interferon and granulocyte colony stimulating factor are in clinical trials. They spur dormant cells to proliferate, thereby forcing stem cells into a division cycle and increasing their sensitivity to chemotherapy. Plexixafor is a stromal cell derived factor which mobilizes stem cells in combination with GCSF which exhibits an anti-metastatic effect. Histone deacetylase inhibitors help to target dormant cells by inducing apoptosis in nonproliferating cancer cell lines and is currently undergoing trial in the study of CML. Valproic acid has been shown to induce tumor cell apoptosis and down regulate EGFR in HNSCC. Finally, Vitamin A derivatives are under investigation for their apparent ability to limit the progression of HNSCC, however effects have been limited to the duration of treatment [26].

Targeting of the EMT pathway focuses on the activated cell signal pathways associated with the mesenchymal transition, such as Wnt/B catenin, PIK3/AKT, MAPK ,and Notch, as well as protein modulators of EMT, such as SNAL. Notch is inhibited by gamma secretase inhibitor mesoporous silica nanoparticles which inhibits cell proliferation and induces apoptosis. Wnt pathway targets include the Wnt proteins themselves, as well as their receptors. Decreasing Wnt signaling decreases the ability of a CSC to maintain the pluripotent state, inhibits proliferation, and hinders epithelial mesenchymal transition. The PIK3/AKT pathway is being investigated for its anti-angiogenic potential, but currently there is no conclusive evidence regarding its use as a therapeutic target in HNSCC [26]. The SNAIL family of proteins has also been implicated in the acquisition of a more malignant tumor phenotype, and directly represses the transcription of E-cadherin, triggering the EMT process.

These proteins are being targeted by SNAIL-inhibitors, with Azmi et al. demonstrating both reversal of EMT phenotype and apoptosis in their cell lines [38].

Investigations targeting stem cells based on surface markers have been somewhat limited by the ongoing search for definitive cancer stem cell markers. Damek-Poprawa et al., conjugated a genetically modified cytolethal distending toxin (Cdt) from the periodontal pathogen *Aggregatibacter actinomycetemcomitans* to anti-human CD133 monoclonal antibodies, and were able to inhibit the proliferation of CD133+ cells in vitro, with sparing of normal oral epithelial cells [39]. Depsite the ubiquitous expression of CD44 and its variant isoforms in normal head and neck epithelia, Platt and Szoka reported selective targeting to cancer via the use of macromolecular carriers, which extravasate preferentially to tumor tissue due to increased tumor vasculature permeability and poor lymphatic egress. They reviewed anti-CD44 agents conjugated to hyaluronic acid, and concluded that targeting therapeutic agents to the CD44 receptor is an area of potential for future molecular therapy [40]. As the biomarker profiles of HNSCCs are refined, this area of research promises to offer specific molecular therapeutic targets.

The CSC provides an attractive therapeutic target in HNSCC, but many therapeutic options remain under pre-clinical investigation. Further research will be required to determine both the efficacy and long term effects of anti-CSC regimens.

Conclusion

The recognition of the cancer stem cell as an entity in tumorigenesis has both illuminated the etiology of recalcitrant HNSCC and clouded the future of treatment for these difficult tumors. As more information is gathered regarding biomarkers, our ability to culture and characterize CSCs will improve, as will our understanding of their targetable pathways and features. Certainly, more research is needed to fully characterize cancer stem cell-specific markers and signaling cascades. As these advances are made, we may have the opportunity to offer patients with advanced or recurrent HNSCC an improved prognosis for the first time in decades.

References

[1] Siegel R, Ma J, Zou Z, Jemal A. Cancer statistics, 2014. *CA Cancer J. Clin.* 2014; 64:9.

[2] Albers AE, Chen C. *Crit. Rev. Oncol. Hematol.* 2012 Mar;81(3):224-40.

[3] Prince ME, Sivanandan R. Proc Natl Acad Sci U S A. 2007 Jan 16;104(3):973-8. *Epub.* 2007 Jan 8.

[4] Weinberg, Robert A. *The Biology of Cancer.* New York: Garland Science, 2014.Print.

[5] Nguyen L, Vanner R. Cancer stem cells: an evolving concept. *Nat. Rev. Cancer* 2012;12(2):133-43.

[6] Hanahan D, Weinberg RA. Hallmarks of cancer: the next generation. *Cell* 2011 Mar 4;144(5):646-74.

[7] Krishnamurthy S, Nor JE. Head and neck cancer stem cells. *J. Dent. Res.* 2012 Apr;91(4):334-40.

[8] Pierce GB, Wallace C. Cancer res. 1971 31:127-134.

[9] Schatton T, Frank NY, Frank MH. Identification and targeting of cancer stem cells. *Bioessays* 2009;31:1038-49.

[10] Lapidot T, Sirard C, Vormoor J, et al. A cell inititiating human acute myeloid leukaemia after transplantation SCID mice. *Nature* 1994;367:645-8.

[11] Reya T, Morrison SJ, Clarke MF, Weissman IL. Stem cells, cancer, and cancer stem cells. *Nature* 414:105-111.

[12] Bonnet D, Dick JE. Human acute myeloid leukemia is organized as a hierarchy that originates from a primitive hematopoietic cell. *Nat. Med.* 1997;3:730-7.

[13] Tabor MH, Clay MR, Owen JH, Bradford CR, et al. Head and neck cancer stem cells: the side population. *Laryngoscope* 2011 Mar;121(3):527-33.

[14] Prince ME, Sivanandan A, Kaczorowski GT, et al. Identification of a subpopulation of cells with cancer stem cell properties in head and neck squamous cell carcinoma. *PNAS* 2007;104(3):973-978.

[15] Prince ME, Ailles LE. Cancer stem cell in head and neck squamous cell cancer. *J. Clin. Oncol.* 2008 Jun 10;26(17):2871-5.

[16] Albers AE, Chen C, Koberle B, et al. Stem cells in squamous head and neck cancer. *Crit. Rev. Oncol. Hemato*. 2012 Mar;81(3):224-40.

[17] Borovski T, De Sousa E, Vermeulen L, Medema JP. Cancer stem cell niche: the place to be. *Cancer Res*. 2011 Feb 1;71(3):634-9.

[18] Krishnamurthy S, Dong Z, Vodopyanov D, et al. Endothelial cell-initiated signaling promotes the survival and self-renewal of cancer stem cells. *Cancer Res.* 2010 December 1; 70(23):9969-78.

[19] Fuchs E, Chen T. A matter of life and death: self-renewal in stem cells. *EMBO Rep.* 2013 Jan;14(1):39-48.

[20] Chikamatsu K, Ishii H, Takahashi G, et al. Resistance to apoptosis-inducing stimuli in CD44+ head and neck squamous cell carcinoma cells. *Head Neck*. 2012 Mar;34(3):336-43.

[21] Wang SJ, Wong G, de Heer AM, Xia W, et al. CD44 variant isoforms in head and neck squamous cell carcinoma progression. *Laryngoscope*. 2009 Aug;119(8):1518-30.

[22] Mack B, Gires O. CD44s and CD44v6 expression in head and neck epithelia. *PLoS One*. 2008;3(10):e3360.

[23] Clay MR, Tabor M, Owen JH, et al. Single marker identification of head and neck squamous cell carcinoma cancer stem cells with aldehyde dehydrogenase. *Head Neck.* 2010 Sep;32(9):1195-201.

[24] Sobreiera TJ, Marletaz F, Simoes-Costa M, et al. Structural shifts of aldehyde dehydrogenase enzymes were instrumental for the early evolution of retinoid-depdent axial matterning in metazoans. *Proc. Natl. Acad. Scnie USA*. 108:226-231.

[25] Chen YC, Chen YW, Hsu HS, et al. Aldehyde dehydrogenase 1 is a putative marker for cancer stem cells in head and neck squamous cancer. *Biochem Biophys. Res. Commun.* 2009;385:307-13.

[26] Papagerakis S, Pannone G, Zhen L, et al. Oral epithelial stem cells – implications in normal development and cancer metastasis. *Exp. Cell* Res. 2014 July 15;325(2):111-129.

[27] Chen H, Zhou L, Dout T, Wan G, et al. BMI-1's maintenance of the proliferative capacity of laryngeal cancer stem cells. *Head Neck*. 2011;33:1115-1125.

[28] Chiou SH, Yu CC, Huang CY, et al. Positive correlations of Oct-4 and Nanog in oral cancer stem-like cells and high grade oral squamous cell carcinoma. *Clin. Cancer Res.* 2008; 14:4085-4095.

[29] Huang CF, Xu XR, Wu TF, et al. Correlations of ALDH1, CD44, OCT4, and SOX2 in tongue squamous cell carcinoma and their association with disease progression and prognosis.

[30] Chuthapisith S. Cancer stem cells and chemoresistance. *Cancer Stem Cells Theories and Practice.* Prof Stanley Shostak (Ed.), ISBN: 978-953-307-225-8, InTech, DOI:105772/13789.

[31] Trock BJ, Leonessa F, Clarke R. Multidrug resistance in breast cancer: a meta-analysis of MDR1/gp170 expression and its possible functional significance. *J. Natl. Cancer Inst.* 89:917-931.

[32] Paez-Ribes M, Allen E, Hudock J, et al. Antiangiogenic therapy elicits malignant progression of tumors to increased local invasion and distant metastasis. *Cancer Cell.* 2009 Mar 3;15(3):220-31.

[33] Keunen O, Johansson M, Oudin A, et al. Anti-VEGF treatment reduces blood supply and increases tumor cell invasion in glioblastoma. *Proc. Natl. Acad. Sci. USA.* 2011 Mar 1;108(9):3749-54.

[34] Leong H, Chong, F, Sew P, et al. Targeting Cancer Stem Cell Plasticity Through Modulation of Epidermal Growth Factor and Insulin-like growth factor receptor signaling in head and neck squamous cell cancer. *Stem Cells Transl. Med.* 2014 Sep;3(9):1055-65.

[35] Noguchi K, Katayama K, Sugimoto Y. Human ABC transporter ABCG2/BCRP expression in chemoresistance: basic and clinical perspectives for molecular cancer therapeutics. *Pharmgenomics Pers. Med.* 2014 Feb 5;7:53-64.

[36] Liu KJ, He JH, Su XD, et al. Saracatinib (AZD0530) is a potent modulator of ABCB1-mediated multidrug resistance in vitro and in vivo. *Int. J. Cancer.* 2013 Jan 1;132(1):224-35.

[37] Croker AK, Allan AL. Inhibitio of aldehyde dehydrogenase (ALDH) activity reduces chemotherapy and radiation resistance of stem-like ALDHhiCD44+ human breast cancer cells. *Breast Cancer Res. Treat.* 2012 May;133(1):75-87.

[38] Azmi AS, Bollig-Fischer A, Bao B, et al. Systems analysis reveals a transcriptional reversal of the mesenchymal phenotype induced by SNAIL inhibitor GN-25. *BMC Systems Biology.* 2013;7:85.

[39] Damek-Poprawa M, Volgina A, Korostoff J, et al. Targeted inhibition of CD133+ cells in oral cancer cell lines. *J. Dent. Res.* 2011 May;90(5): 638-645.

[40] Platt V, Szoka F. Anticancer therapeutics: targeting macromolecules and nanocarriers to hyaluronan or CD44, a hyaluronan receptor. *Mol. Pharm.* 2008 Jul-Aug; 5(4): 474-486.

In: Head and Neck Cancer
Editor: Madison R. Hall

ISBN: 978-1-63482-113-1

Chapter 3

The Growing Significance of Human Epidermal Growth Factor Receptor 2 (HER2) As Therapeutic Treatment Target in Head and Neck Cancer

Wei Gao, Thian Sze Wong*, Jie Luo and Jimmy Yuwai Chan
Department of Surgery, Faculty of Medicine,
The University of Hong Kong, Hong Kong

Abstract

Attenuation of the cell surface receptor (epidermal growth factor receptor, EGFR) mediated signaling cascade is a proven effective treatment approach in treating epithelial malignancies. The receptor tyrosine kinase (RTK) could be activated by a number of growth factors reversibly such as EGF, TGF-alpha, heregulins and HB-EGF. Inhibition of the activation of the EGFR receptor will block the activation of significant oncogenic signaling cascades including phosphatidylinositol-3-kinase (PI3K)/AKT pathway, mitogen-activated protein kinase (MAPK) pathway and JAK-STAT signaling pathway. Aberrations of the EGFR family are frequently observed in head and neck cancer. Specific genotypes will affect the treatment outcome and hence impact the prognosis of cancer patients. The use of EGFR tyrosine kinase inhibitors or specific antibodies is proven to be useful. However, the effects will gradually decline with the development of resistant phenotype. Recent data suggest that cancer cells will compensate the loss of EGFR-mediated signaling effects by increasing the signaling output of other EGFR members such as HER2. Human HER2 (ERBB2 or NEU) is one of the 4 members of the EGFR family. Gene amplification and protein overexpression of HER2 are found in head and neck cancer. Histological data revealed that protein overexpression of HER2 is site-specific with particular high frequency observed in a subset of cancers in head and neck regions. This chapter will provide a summary on HER2 with particular focus on the

* Corresponding author: Thian Sze Wong. E-mail: thiansze@gmail.com.

therapeutic aspects. Further, the significance of HER2 and the growing recognition of the particular functional roles in head and neck cancers will be addressed.

1. Introduction

Cancer is a major public health issue and is a major cause of death. Due to the aging population structure worldwide, it is likely that the burden will increase progressively. Most of the human cancers (up to 85%) are originated from epithelial cells. Epithelial cancer could be derived from different cell types in the epithelial layers covering the outside body and inner organs including squamous cell, adenomatous cells, and transitional cells.

Development of effective target treatment regime which acts on specific oncogenic gene/protein in the epithelial cancers is one of the greatest challenges in therapeutic medicine. The epithelial cancer cell has an inappropriately high proliferation rate in comparison with the normal counterparts. This is achieved by overexpressing the epithelial cell specific growth factor receptors. Once stimulated or activated by growth factor ligands, pro-tumorigenic signals will be delivered which later drives the development of cancerous phenotype. Different from the conventional therapeutic regime such as chemotherapy which deliver chemical compounds to the cancer sites to reverse the disease stages, tailored treatment with the use of targeted therapeutic agent has high selectivity against for tumor cells with limited toxic side effects. Hence, there is significant paradigm shift of the anti-cancer drug developmental process in recent years, which focus on specific target gene or gene products.

Human epidermal growth factor receptor (EGFR) family is a class of well-validated oncogenic marker for epithelial cancers. The EGFR family is receptor protein.

The tyrosine kinase complexes expresses on the cell surface of the epithelial cells. The family has 4 members including ERBB1 (HER1 or EGFR), ERBB2 (HER2 and NEU), ERBB3 (HER3) and ERBB4 (HER4). Activation of the EGFR family receptors is achieved by phosphorylation of the receptor resulting in a significant amplification of the growth promoting and survival signals. ERBB2 overexpression is documented in a number of human epithelial cancers (Martin, Cappuzzo, Mazzucchelli, and Frattini, 2014). The oncogenic effects of ERBB2 and the causal relationship with cancer development are conclusive with the use of animal models (Ursini-Siegel, Schade, Cardiff, and Muller, 2007). ERBB2 could form dimers with the other 3 EGFR family members (HER1, HER3 and HER4) leading to the formation of functional receptors on the cancer cell surface (Moasser, 2014). Although there are several FDA-approved ERBB2 inhibitors available, increasing data suggested that the inhibitor developed in the 80's could not completely attenuate the constitutively active ERBB2 signaling cascade in cancer cells (Moasser, 2014). Apart from the direct cancer promoting functions, recent findings indicate that ERBB2 is involved in the development of resistant cancer phenotypes against the treatment agents. It is recognized that monotherapy against the EGFR receptors (especially ERBB1) is only effective at the beginning treatment stages. In many cases, development of resistance will occur because the cancer cells will try to maintain and preserve the signal throughput and bypass the inhibition through overpowering the signal output from other EGFR family members (Moasser, 2014). The idea is supported by the observation that concurrently targeting two or more EGFR family members could yield a higher therapeutic effect in the cancer patients (Huang et al., 2013).

Hence, there is a pressing need to develop novel therapeutic modulations targeting other EGFR members in order to perfect the current treatment regime against the EGFR family.

2. Structure, Function, Gene Amplification and Protein Expression of HER2

HER2 was firstly found in embryonic fibroblasts of mouse and was named as oncogene neu (Shih, Padhy, Murray, and Weinberg, 1981). In carcinogen-stimulated rat neuro/glioblastomas, neu was found to be activated, which firstly implicated that HER2 may play a crucial role in cancer (Schechter et al., 1984). HRE2 is a receptor tyrosine kinase with the molecular weight of 185 kDa. The domain structure of HER2 consists of an intracellular kinase domain with catalytic activity and an extracellular domain. HER2 exhibits higher catalytic kinase activity than other three EGFR family members. HER2 does not harbor a ligand-binding domain that has been found in other family proteins, making it a unique member among the family (T. P. Garrett et al., 2003). For other family receptors, the binding of ligand results in a change in conformation allowing the generation of homo- and hetero-dimers. In contrast, no ligands have been demonstrated to interact with HER2. However, the extracellular domain of HER2 shows an active conformation independent of the presence of any ligands, which favors its dimerization with other family receptors (T. P. Garrett et al., 2003). Therefore, HER2 acts as a signal amplifier of other family receptors via the formation of heterodimers between them (Arkhipov, Shan, Kim, Dror, and Shaw, 2013). Since the heterodimers containing HER2 are frequently recycled to the cell surface and HER2 is able to suppress the dissociation rate of ligand, HER2 becomes the most active dimerization partner and receptor heterodimers harboring HER2 represent the signaling complex with the strongest activity among the whole family (Lenferink et al., 1998; Tzahar et al., 1996).

2.1. Heterodimers of HER2

Although HER2 could form heterodimers with EGFR, HER3 and HER4, it generates signal particularly through HER3 (Holbro, Beerli, et al., 2003). The binding of ligand to HER3 leads to reconfiguration of its extracellular domain, which mediates the production of dimers with HER2. HER3 stimulated by ligand is preferred to bind HER2 (Alimandi et al., 1995). Subsequently, the kinase domain of HER3 activates the kinase domain of HER2, which in turn results in the phosphorylation of c-tail of HER3. Finally, this process leads to the recruitment of a number of proteins and promotes a wide variety of signaling cascades (Alimandi et al., 1995). In addition, enhanced expression of HER2 increases the heterodimerization between HER2 and HER3 (Yarden and Sliwkowski, 2001).

2.2. Downstream Signaling Pathways of HER2

The downstream signaling pathways of HER2 include phosphatidylinositide-3 kinase (PI3K)/AKT and MAPK signaling pathways.

HER2 activates various downstream signaling pathways through heterodimerization with HER3 or EGFR. HER2 and EGFR heterodimers are preferred to promote MAPK signaling, whereas HER2 and HER3 heterodimers preferentially stimulate PI3K/AKT pathway (Holbro, Civenni, and Hynes, 2003). In HER2-driven human cancers, HER3 but not EGFR is frequently phosphorylated and activated as evidenced by the observation that knockout of HER3 but not EGFR suppresses cell viability (Lee-Hoeflich et al., 2008). Although HER2 could not directly stimulate PI3K/AKT, it exerts its function via activation of its heterodimer partner HER3. Silence of HER3 or an antibody neutralizing HER3 suppresses tumor growth of HER2-driven xenograft, indicating that HER3 is necessary for HER2-amplified tumor (J. T. Garrett et al., 2013).

2.3. Gene Amplification, Protein Overexpression and Mutation of HER2

The expression patterns of HER2 are classified into HER2-negative tumors with normal HER2 expression level and HER2-positive tumors with HER2 amplification and overexpression. Amplification of HER2 gene leads to overexpression of its protein. Immunohistochemistry (IHC) is employed to measure the protein expression level of HER2 and fluorescence in situ hybridization (FISH) is used to evaluate amplification of HER2 gene (Wolff et al., 2007). The use of different detection methods and various evaluation criteria cause inaccuracy in assessment of HER2 status. Therefore, the College of American Pathologists (CAP) and the American Society of Clinical Oncology (ASCO) generated a guideline to direct the test and interpretation of HER2 status in 2007, aiming to minimize the variation derived from different laboratories (Wolff et al., 2007). In the guideline, the thresholds of protein expression level and the ratios of gene copy were defined for HER2. Gene amplification or protein overexpression of HER2 was found in a various percentage of cancer cases, such as approximately 20% of breast cancer, 20% of gastric cancer, 5–15% of bladder cancer, 1–21% of cervix cancer, 2–3% of colorectal cancer, 4–22% of esophageal cancer, 7–15% of glioblastoma, 2.4% of liver cancer, 1–6% of non-small cell lung cancer, 6–7% of ovarian cancer and 2–29% of pancreatic cancer (Yan, Parker, Schwab, and Kurzrock, 2014). Gene amplification and overexpression of HER2 are correlated with a poor prognosis of cancer patients (Slamon et al., 1989). A number of methods have been employed to detect HER2 mutations such as sequenom analysis, single-strand conformational polymorphism depending on PCR as well as next generation sequencing. A small proportion of cancer cases harbor somatic HER2 mutations (Arteaga and Engelman, 2014). These mutations are found in breast cancer, lung cancer, gastric cancer, bladder cancer, and endometrial cancer. The majority of these mutations are missense mutations located at the extracellular domain and tyrosine kinase domain (Arteaga and Engelman, 2014). Furthermore, HER2 mutations are not present in cancers with gene amplification. Several mutations result in activated signal of HER2.

3. The Significance of HER2 in Head and Neck Cancer Treatment

In head and neck cancer, results from IHC showed that HER2 was overexpressed in a variable proportion of tumor samples ranging from 7-76% (Ali et al., 2010; Azemar et al., 2000; Cavalot et al., 2007; Khademi et al., 2002). In laryngeal carcinoma, HER2 overexpression was found in 10.5-68% tumor samples by IHC (Khademi et al., 2002; Wei et al., 2008). HER2 was overexpressed in 51% cases of patients with oral cancer (Xia et al., 1997). Although a number of studies carried out IHC to detect the protein expression level of HER2 in head and neck cancer, only one study performed FISH to assess its gene amplification. Results from FISH demonstrated that HER2 amplification was found in 3.6% cases (Freier et al., 2003). Cavalot et al. revealed that high expression level of HER2 was positively associated with capsule rupture, lymph node metastasis, and vascular embolization in head and neck cancer (Cavalot et al., 2007). In addition, patients with high HER2 expression exhibited a shorter overall survival (OS) and disease-free survival (DFS) compared with patients with low expression level (Cavalot et al., 2007). Moreover, protein expression level of HER2 could serve as an independent prognostic factor for DFS. Likewise, Xia et al. also demonstrated that high expression level of HER2 was positively correlated with lymph node metastasis, distant metastasis as well as poor overall survival in oral cancer (Xia et al., 1997). On the contrary, two independent studies showed that HER2 expression level was not associated with any clinicopathological parameters including tumor size, lymph node metastasis, sex, age and survival (Ali et al., 2010; Sardari et al., 2012).

HER2 was shown to be expressed in the same areas as EGFR in almost all cases of oropharyngeal squamous cell carcinomas, implicating the co-expression between them (Ibrahim et al., 1999). Likewise, Khademi et al. also reported that HER2 and EGFR were co-expressed in 68% tumor samples from patients with head and neck cancer (Khademi et al., 2002). The expression of HER2 was positively associated with activated HER2 (phosphorylated HER2) and EGFR by analysis of 213 tumors of head and neck cancer in TCPA database (The Cancer Proteome Atlas) (Pollock and Grandis, 2014). To investigate the mechanisms underlying the acquired resistance to cetuximab which targets EGFR, the in vivo resistant model was generated by treating sensitive xenogragt with increasing doses of cetuximab and the resistance was confirmed by invasion assay (Quesnelle and Grandis, 2011). In head and neck cancer cells resistant to cetuximab, the C-terminal of HER2 displayed enhanced phosphorylation, suggesting that co-expression or activation of HER2 with EGFR might contribute to the resistance to treatment towards EGFR. The combination of cetuximab with afatinib, which is a kinase inhibitor towards both EGFR and HER2, generated a synergistic effect on the inhibition of cell growth, which further confirmed that the resistance to cetuximab was attributed to co-overexpression or activation of HER2 in head and neck cancer (Quesnelle and Grandis, 2011).

4. Specific Drugs Targeting HER2

4.1. Monoclonal Antibodies

Trastuzumab is an antibody which could bind to the juxtamembrane region in the extracellular domain of HER2 receptor. It unravels the heterodimer containing HER2 through suppression of the cleavage of extracellular domain inside HER2, leading to suppression of its intracellular kinase activity and downstream cascades (Ghosh et al., 2011). In addition, it triggers cytotoxicity dependent on antibody and promotes endocytosis of HER2, resulting in lysis of tumor (Hudis, 2007). Moreover, trastuzumab mediates an adaptive immune response via recruiting T cells to eradicate tumor as evidenced by the observation that mice deficient in macrophages and natural killer cells displayed significantly reduced response to trastuzumab treatment (Clynes, Towers, Presta, and Ravetch, 2000). Trastuzumab is the first approved drug targeting HER2 to treat advanced gastric cancer as well as breast cancer with metastasis (Bang et al., 2010; Romond et al., 2005). Pertuzumab is an antibody which interacts with heterodimerization domain II in HER2, leading to inhibition of dimerization between HER2 and HER3 and sequential suppression of PI3K/AKT pathway (Agus et al., 2002). Pertuzumab combined with trastuzumab and docetaxel elevated response rate and progression-free survival in breast cancer setting in comparison with trastuzumab and docetaxel alone, suggesting that various but complementary mechanisms underlying the anti-HRE2 effects of pertuzumab and trastuzumab contributed to the synergistic clinical efficiency (Baselga et al., 2012; Gianni et al., 2012). Although trastuzumab and pertuzumab alone showed limited inhibitory effects as a monotherapy reagent, they indeed improved the therapeutic efficiency of chemotherapy modality in the treatment of advanced gastric and breast cancers (Baselga et al., 2012; Slamon et al., 2001). The synergistic effect of trastuzumab and pertuzumab with chemotherapy was more significant for early-stage breast cancer as shown by a longer survival.

In head and neck cancer, pertuzumab combined with gefitinib was explored in cell line model in vitro. Head and neck cancer cells resistant to gefitinib, a tyrosine kinase inhibitor targeting EGFR, exhibited elevated levels of phosphorylated HER2. Pertuzumab combined with gefitinib generated additive inhibitory effects on cell growth in comparison with gefitinib alone, indicating that inactivation of HER2 by pertuzumab overcame resistance to gefitinib (Erjala et al., 2006). In addition, although trastuzumab enhanced the efficacy of chemotherapeutic reagents in gastric and breast cancers, a phase II clinical trial revealed that trastuzumab combined with paclitaxel and cisplatin did not elevate the response rate of head and neck cancer patient to chemotherapy management.

4.2. Tyrosine Kinase Inhibitors

4.2.1. Lapatinib

Lapatinib is a reversible dual tyrosine kinase inhibitor targeting both HER2 and EGFR (Konecny et al., 2006). It is approved by FDA to treat breast cancer with positive HER2 status. Lapatinib inhibits HER2 and EGFR by competing with ATP in interacting with the kinase domain, thus suppressing their tyrosine kinase activity. Lapatinib efficiently suppresses HER2 and downstream PI3K/AKT and MAPK signaling cascades in breast cancer, leading to induction of apoptosis and inhibition of cell proliferation and growth. It exhibits improved clinical efficacy than trastuzumab (Geyer et al., 2006). Therefore, lapatinib is employed to treat patients with breast cancer who have relapsed from a first-line management using modality containing trastuzumab.

Moreover, lapatinib is preferred to be used in combination with trastuzumab or capecitabine to improve clinical efficiency (Blackwell et al., 2012).

In head and neck cancer, the therapeutic effects of lapatinib in combination with cisplatin were evaluated in an ex vivo model (Schrader et al., 2012). The biopsies of head and neck cancer were treated by a series of lapatinib dilutions following grind and collagenase digestion. The addition of lapatinib improved the therapeutic efficacy of cisplatin as shown by colony formation assays. Nevertheless, a significant inter-individual variation was found in the concentration of lapatinib required for inhibition of colony formation to 50%, implicating that head and neck cancers harbored a pronounced heterogeneity in response to lapatinib treatment. Similarly, another study assessed the anti-cancer activity of lapatinib in combination with cisplatin or paclitaxel in head and neck cancer cell lines both in vitro and in vivo (Kondo et al., 2010). In vitro experiments demonstrated that lapatinib suppressed cell growth, whereas the anti-proliferation effects of lapatinib was not associated with the expression of HER2. In vivo studies revealed that lapatinib enhanced the induction of apoptosis in xenograft derived from YCU-H891 cells in nude mice, suggesting its anti-tumor effects. Although lapatinib alone could not suppress angiogenesis, the combination of lapatinib with paclitaxel significantly inhibited angiogenesis and triggered apoptosis. Overall, these findings indicated that lapatinib combined with cisplatin yielded synergistic effects on head and neck cancer cells (Kondo et al., 2010).

4.2.2. Afatinib

Afatinib is irreversible tyrosine kinase inhibitor that could target EGFR family receptors including HER2, HER4, and EGFR via binding to their tyrosine kinase domain (Solca et al., 2012). Since afatinib covalently interacts with kinase domain, it irreversibly suppresses signaling from EGFR receptors. A phase III clinical trial revealed that afatinib treatment resulted in a significant improvement of progression-free survival of patients with EGFR-mutated lung cancer when compared to chemotherapy (Sequist et al., 2013). Based on this promising result, afatinib is approved by FDA to treat patients with non-small cell lung cancer who contain mutant forms of EGFR. Recently, three patients who failed in treatment regime containing anti-EGFR and anti-HER2 reagents exhibited objective response to afatinib, further supporting its beneficial effects on patients (De Greve et al., 2012). The encouraging results on the use of afatinib derived from non-small cell lung cancer have promoted the studies in head and neck cancer. Afatinib treatment led to a pronounced inhibition of xenograft tumor derived from FaDu (hypopharyngeal cancer cell line) cells in mice (Harbeck, Solca, and Gauler, 2014).

4.2.3. Dacomitinib

Dacomitinib (PF00299804) is an irreversible EGFR and HER2 tyrosine kinase inhibitor (Engelman et al., 2007). Dacomitinib not only targeted wild-type EGFR and HER2, but also inhibited their mutation forms. In non-small cell lung cancers, gefitinib and erlotinib could effectively suppress tumor growth. Nevertheless, despite of good initial response, cancers will unavoidably develop resistance due to secondary EGFR mutation such as T790M. Dacomitinib could inhibit T790M mutation of EGFR both in vitro and in vivo in non-small cell lung cancers. Moreover, dacomitinib also targeted HER2 mutation occurred in lung cancer with high efficiency (Engelman et al., 2007). The efficacy of dacomitinib alone or in combination with radiation was also assessed in both head and neck cancer cell line model and mice model (Williams et al., 2014). Dacomitinib treatment suppressed the cell viability and colony formation ability in a dose-dependent manner in three head and neck cancer cell line (UT-SCC-8, FaDu, and UT-SCC-42a). Dacomitinib also inhibited tumor growth of xenograft derived from FaDu (Williams et al., 2014). The EGFR and downstream signaling cascades such as ERK, AKT as well as mTOR pathway were inhibited by dacomitinib treatment. Nevertheless, the effects of dacomitinib on HER2 signaling should be investigated in future. Dacomitinib combined with radiation generated synergistic effects on the inhibition of cell viability and tumor growth in both cell lines and mouse xenograft models, supporting further assessment of dacomitinib in combination with radiotherapy to manage patients with head and neck cancer in clinical trials (Williams et al., 2014).

5. Clinical Trials on HER2 in Head and Neck Cancer

Encouraging results obtained from preclinical studies have promoted a wide variety of clinical trials on the therapeutic effects of HER2 inhibitor alone or combined with other reagent for the management of head and neck cancer.

Most of these clinical trials listed in ClinicalTrials.gov are ongoing and recruiting patients. Several studies have reported the efficacy of HER2 inhibitors.

The therapeutic effects of the use of lapatinib before chemoradiotherapy were evaluated in 107 patients with locally advanced head and neck cancers in a phase II clinical trials (Del Campo et al., 2011). Patients were administrated with lapatinib or placebo for 4 weeks followed by chemoradiotherapy. Lapatinib treatment significantly reduced the proliferation of tumor as shown by Ki67 assay in comparison with placebo. However, lapatinib treatment did not enhance apoptosis when compared to placebo. Lapatinib monotherapy indeed resulted in a better objective response rate (17%) than that (0%) of placebo alone. Among these patients who respond to lapatinib, all exhibited overexpression of EGFR and half of them displayed overexpression of HER2. However, these patients showed high heterogeneity in response to lapatinib in term of proliferation, apoptosis as well as EGFR phosphorylation (Del Campo et al., 2011). Administration of lapatinib also yielded side effects such as odynophagia, dysphagia, and mucosal inflammation. Lapatinib combined with chemoradiotherapy also exhibited improved objective response rate (70%) in comparison with the combination of placebo and chemoradiotherapy (53%). Although the difference did not reach statistical significance, the improvement warranted further study on lapatinib using a larger sample size.

The efficacy and safety of lapatinib as monotherapy was assessed in patients with recurrent or metastatic head and neck cancer by de Souza et al. (de Souza et al., 2012). In this study, patients were divided into two groups depending on with or without former treatment by EGFR inhibitor. Biological effects of lapatinib were evaluated by IHC staining of EGFR and HER2 in matched tumor samples before and after treatment. EGFR and HER2 were expressed in most patients and lapatinib treatment significantly reduced the pHER2/HER2 ratio but not phosphorylation of EGFR and downstream signaling such as ERK and AKT (de Souza et al., 2012). In most patients, lapatinib generated grade 1 or grade 2 toxicities such as diarrhea and rash and did not cause treatment-associated death. Although lapatinib treatment did not cause severe side effects, lapatinib monotherapy did not benefit either EGFR inhibitor-naive or resistant patients as evidenced by the fact that no partial or complete responses were found in both groups (de Souza et al., 2012).

Two clinical trials revealed that afatinib monotherapy indeed benefited patients with recurrent or metastatic head and neck cancer. The anti-cancer properties of afatinib were compared with cetuximab, which is the only FDA-approved targeting therapy reagent for head and neck cancer.

Afatinib yielded anti-cancer activity comparable to cetuximab as evidenced by even better tumor shrinkage and objective response rate as well as similar disease control rates. Nevertheless, adverse events such as rash/ acne, diarrhea, and stomatitis/mucositis were more frequent in afatinib group than those in cetuximab group, resulting in a higher treatment discontinuation rate in afatinib group. Another completed phase III trial (NCT01345682) demonstrated that afatinib administration resulted in beneficial effects on patients with recurrent or metastatic head and neck cancer when compared to methotrexate (Pollock and Grandis, 2014). Afatinib treatment significantly enhanced progress-free survival, objective response rate as well as disease control rate in comparison with methotrexate (Pollock and Grandis, 2014).

Conclusion

HER2 exhibits the highest catalytic kinase activity and it shows a constitutively active conformation independent of ligands, which make HER2 a unique member among the EGFR family receptors. HER2 is the most active dimerization partner due to the frequent recycling of HER2-containing heterodimers to the cell surface and the inhibitory effects of HER2 on the dissociation rate of ligand. Overall, HER2-harboring receptor heterodimers show the highest activity among the whole family, suggesting that HER2 is a promising therapeutic target. Overexpression of HER2 protein due to gene amplification of HER2 gene as well as activating mutations of HER2 stimulates downstream signaling cascades including PI3K/AKT and MAPK pathway. Overexpression of HER2 protein is frequently found in head and neck cancer, however, gene amplification and mutations of HER2 are relative less reported, which is partial attributed to less studies on them. To investigate the mechanisms underlying the overexpression of HER2 and identify activating HER2 mutations for personalized therapy, further studies on gene amplification and mutations of HER2 are needed. High protein expression levels of HER2 are well associated with lymph node metastasis, distant metastasis as well as poor overall survival, implicating the prognostic value of HER2.

HER2 is co-expressed with EGFR in almost all cases of head and neck cancer and activation of HER2 confers resistance to cetuximab, the only FDA-approved targeting therapy reagent for head and neck cancer. Preclinical study reveals that afatinib, a dual inhibitor of EGFR and HER2, generates synergistic inhibitory effects with cetuximab in cell line model.

Likewise, pertuzumab combined with gefitinib leads to additive inhibitory effects on cell growth. These findings demonstrate that combination of EGFR inhibitor and HER2 inhibitor results in synergistic effects. Since tumor will develop resistance to a reagent targeting only one molecule, most clinical trials carried out in head and neck cancer focus on inhibitors that dually target EGFR and HER2 including lapatinib and afatinib. Although clinical trials reveal that lapatinib or afatinib monotherapy indeed benefits patients with recurrent or metastatic head and neck cancer, the therapeutic effects are still limited. Therefore, combination of these inhibitors with chemotherapy, radiotherapy or chemoradiotherapy should be investigated in future aiming to obtain the maximum beneficial effects for patients.

References

Agus, D. B., Akita, R. W., Fox, W. D., Lewis, G. D., Higgins, B., Pisacane, P. I., ... Sliwkowski, M. X. (2002). Targeting ligand-activated ErbB2 signaling inhibits breast and prostate tumor growth. *Cancer Cell,* 2(2), 127-137.

Ali, M. A., Gunduz, M., Gunduz, E., Tamamura, R., Beder, L. B., Katase, N., ... Nagatsuka, H. (2010). Expression and mutation analysis of her2 in head and neck squamous cell carcinoma. *Cancer Invest.,* 28(5), 495-500. doi: 10.3109/07357900903476778.

Alimandi, M., Romano, A., Curia, M. C., Muraro, R., Fedi, P., Aaronson, S. A., ... Kraus, M. H. (1995). Cooperative signaling of ErbB3 and ErbB2 in neoplastic transformation and human mammary carcinomas. *Oncogene,* 10(9), 1813-1821.

Arkhipov, A., Shan, Y., Kim, E. T., Dror, R. O., and Shaw, D. E. (2013). Her2 activation mechanism reflects evolutionary preservation of asymmetric ectodomain dimers in the human EGFR family. *Elife,* 2, e00708. doi: 10. 7554/eLife.00708.

Arteaga, C. L. and Engelman, J. A. (2014). ERBB receptors: from oncogene discovery to basic science to mechanism-based cancer therapeutics. *Cancer Cell,* 25(3), 282-303. doi: 10.1016/j.ccr.2014.02.025.

Azemar, M., Schmidt, M., Arlt, F., Kennel, P., Brandt, B., Papadimitriou, A., ... Wels, W. (2000). Recombinant antibody toxins specific for ErbB2 and EGF receptor inhibit the in vitro growth of human head and neck cancer cells and cause rapid tumor regression in vivo. *Int. J. Cancer,* 86(2), 269-275.

Bang, Y. J., Van Cutsem, E., Feyereislova, A., Chung, H. C., Shen, L., Sawaki, A., ... Kang, Y. K. (2010). Trastuzumab in combination with chemotherapy versus chemotherapy alone for treatment of HER2-positive advanced gastric or gastro-oesophageal junction cancer (ToGA): a phase 3, open-label, randomised controlled trial. *Lancet,* 376(9742), 687-697. doi: 10.1016/s0140-6736(10)61121-x.

Baselga, J., Cortes, J., Kim, S. B., Im, S. A., Hegg, R., Im, Y. H., ... Swain, S. M. (2012). Pertuzumab plus trastuzumab plus docetaxel for metastatic breast cancer. *N. Engl. J. Med.,* 366(2), 109-119. doi: 10.1056/NEJMoa 1113216.

Blackwell, K. L., Burstein, H. J., Storniolo, A. M., Rugo, H. S., Sledge, G., Aktan, G., ... O'Shaughnessy, J. (2012). Overall survival benefit with lapatinib in combination with trastuzumab for patients with human epidermal growth factor receptor 2-positive metastatic breast cancer: final results from the EGF104900 Study. *J. Clin. Oncol.,* 30(21), 2585-2592. doi: 10.1200/jco.2011.35.6725.

Cavalot, A., Martone, T., Roggero, N., Brondino, G., Pagano, M., and Cortesina, G. (2007). Prognostic impact of HER-2/neu expression on squamous head and neck carcinomas. *Head Neck,* 29(7), 655-664. doi: 10. 1002/hed.20574.

Clynes, R. A., Towers, T. L., Presta, L. G., and Ravetch, J. V. (2000). Inhibitory Fc receptors modulate in vivo cytotoxicity against tumor targets. *Nat. Med.,* 6(4), 443-446. doi: 10.1038/74704.

De Greve, J., Teugels, E., Geers, C., Decoster, L., Galdermans, D., De Mey, J., ... Schallier, D. (2012). Clinical activity of afatinib (BIBW 2992) in patients with lung adenocarcinoma with mutations in the kinase domain of HER2/neu. *Lung Cancer,* 76(1), 123-127. doi: 10.1016/j.lungcan.2012.01. 008.

De Souza, J. A., Davis, D. W., Zhang, Y., Khattri, A., Seiwert, T. Y., Aktolga, S., ... Cohen, E. E. (2012). A phase II study of lapatinib in recurrent/ metastatic squamous cell carcinoma of the head and neck. *Clin. Cancer Res.,* 18(8), 2336-2343. doi: 10.1158/1078-0432.ccr-11-2825.

Del Campo, J. M., Hitt, R., Sebastian, P., Carracedo, C., Lokanatha, D., Bourhis, J., ... Harrington, K. J. (2011). Effects of lapatinib monotherapy: results of a randomised phase II study in therapy-naive patients with locally advanced squamous cell carcinoma of the head and neck. *Br. J. Cancer,* 105(5), 618-627. doi: 10.1038/bjc.2011.237.

Engelman, J. A., Zejnullahu, K., Gale, C. M., Lifshits, E., Gonzales, A. J., Shimamura, T., ... Janne, P. A. (2007). PF00299804, an irreversible pan-ERBB inhibitor, is effective in lung cancer models with EGFR and ERBB2 mutations that are resistant to gefitinib. *Cancer Res.,* 67(24), 11924-11932. doi: 10.1158/0008-5472.can-07-1885.

Erjala, K., Sundvall, M., Junttila, T. T., Zhang, N., Savisalo, M., Mali, P., ... Elenius, K. (2006). Signaling via ErbB2 and ErbB3 associates with resistance and epidermal growth factor receptor (EGFR) amplification with sensitivity to EGFR inhibitor gefitinib in head and neck squamous cell carcinoma cells. *Clin. Cancer Res.,* 12(13), 4103-4111. doi: 10.1158/ 1078-0432.ccr-05-2404.

Freier, K., Joos, S., Flechtenmacher, C., Devens, F., Benner, A., Bosch, F. X., ... Hofele, C. (2003). Tissue microarray analysis reveals site-specific prevalence of oncogene amplifications in head and neck squamous cell carcinoma. *Cancer Res.,* 63(6), 1179-1182.

Garrett, J. T., Sutton, C. R., Kurupi, R., Bialucha, C. U., Ettenberg, S. A., Collins, S. D., ... Arteaga, C. L. (2013). Combination of antibody that inhibits ligand-independent HER3 dimerization and a p110alpha inhibitor potently blocks PI3K signaling and growth of HER2+ breast cancers. *Cancer Res.,* 73(19), 6013-6023. doi: 10.1158/0008-5472.can-13-1191.

Garrett, T. P., McKern, N. M., Lou, M., Elleman, T. C., Adams, T. E., Lovrecz, G. O., ... Ward, C. W. (2003). The crystal structure of a truncated ErbB2 ectodomain reveals an active conformation, poised to interact with other ErbB receptors. *Mol. Cell,* 11(2), 495-505.

Geyer, C. E., Forster, J., Lindquist, D., Chan, S., Romieu, C. G., Pienkowski, T., ... Cameron, D. (2006). Lapatinib plus capecitabine for HER2-positive advanced breast cancer. *N. Engl. J. Med.,* 355(26), 2733-2743. doi: 10. 1056/NEJMoa064320.

Ghosh, R., Narasanna, A., Wang, S. E., Liu, S., Chakrabarty, A., Balko, J. M., ... Arteaga, C. L. (2011). Trastuzumab has preferential activity against breast cancers driven by HER2 homodimers. *Cancer Res.,* 71(5), 1871-1882. doi: 10.1158/0008-5472.can-10-1872.

Gianni, L., Pienkowski, T., Im, Y. H., Roman, L., Tseng, L. M., Liu, M. C., ... Valagussa, P. (2012). Efficacy and safety of neoadjuvant pertuzumab and trastuzumab in women with locally advanced, inflammatory, or early HER2-positive breast cancer (NeoSphere): a randomised multicentre, open-label, phase 2 trial. *Lancet Oncol.,* 13(1), 25-32. doi: 10.1016/s1470-2045(11)70336-9.

Harbeck, N., Solca, F. and Gauler, T. C. (2014). Preclinical and clinical development of afatinib: a focus on breast cancer and squamous cell carcinoma of the head and neck. *Future Oncol.,* 10(1), 21-40. doi: 10. 2217/fon.13.244.

Holbro, T., Beerli, R. R., Maurer, F., Koziczak, M., Barbas, C. F., 3rd, and Hynes, N. E. (2003). The ErbB2/ErbB3 heterodimer functions as an oncogenic unit: ErbB2 requires ErbB3 to drive breast tumor cell proliferation. *Proc. Natl. Acad. Sci. US,* 100(15), 8933-8938. doi: 10.1073 /pnas.1537685100.

Holbro, T., Civenni, G. and Hynes, N. E. (2003). The ErbB receptors and their role in cancer progression. *Exp. Cell Res.,* 284(1), 99-110.

Huang, S., Li, C., Armstrong, E. A., Peet, C. R., Saker, J., Amler, L. C., ... Harari, P. M. (2013). Dual targeting of EGFR and HER3 with MEHD7945A overcomes acquired resistance to EGFR inhibitors and radiation. *Cancer Res.,* 73(2), 824-833. doi: 10.1158/0008-5472.can-12-1611.

Hudis, C. A. (2007). Trastuzumab--mechanism of action and use in clinical practice. *N. Engl. J. Med.,* 357(1), 39-51. doi: 10.1056/NEJMra043186.

Ibrahim, S. O., Lillehaug, J. R., Johannessen, A. C., Liavaag, P. G., Nilsen, R., and Vasstrand, E. N. (1999). Expression of biomarkers (p53, transforming growth factor alpha, epidermal growth factor receptor, c-erbB-2/neu and the proliferative cell nuclear antigen) in oropharyngeal squamous cell carcinomas. *Oral Oncol.,* 35(3), 302-313.

Khademi, B., Shirazi, F. M., Vasei, M., Doroudchi, M., Gandomi, B., Modjtahedi, H., ... Ghaderi, A. (2002). The expression of p53, c-erbB-1 and c-erbB-2 molecules and their correlation with prognostic markers in patients with head and neck tumors. *Cancer Lett.,* 184(2), 223-230.

Kondo, N., Tsukuda, M., Ishiguro, Y., Kimura, M., Fujita, K., Sakakibara, A., ... Matsuda, H. (2010). Antitumor effects of lapatinib (GW572016), a dual inhibitor of EGFR and HER-2, in combination with cisplatin or paclitaxel on head and neck squamous cell carcinoma. *Oncol. Rep.,* 23(4), 957-963.

Konecny, G. E., Pegram, M. D., Venkatesan, N., Finn, R., Yang, G., Rahmeh, M., ... Slamon, D. J. (2006). Activity of the dual kinase inhibitor lapatinib (GW572016) against HER-2-overexpressing and trastuzumab-treated breast cancer cells. *Cancer Res.,* 66(3), 1630-1639. doi: 10.1158/0008-5472.can-05-1182.

Lee-Hoeflich, S. T., Crocker, L., Yao, E., Pham, T., Munroe, X., Hoeflich, K. P., ... Stern, H. M. (2008). A central role for HER3 in HER2-amplified breast cancer: implications for targeted therapy. *Cancer Res.,* 68(14), 5878-5887. doi: 10.1158/0008-5472.can-08-0380.

Lenferink, A. E., Pinkas-Kramarski, R., van de Poll, M. L., van Vugt, M. J., Klapper, L. N., Tzahar, E., ... Yarden, Y. (1998). Differential endocytic routing of homo- and hetero-dimeric ErbB tyrosine kinases confers signaling superiority to receptor heterodimers. *Embo J.,* 17(12), 3385-3397. doi: 10.1093/emboj/17.12.3385.

Martin, V., Cappuzzo, F., Mazzucchelli, L., and Frattini, M. (2014). HER2 in solid tumors: more than 10 years under the microscope; where are we now? *Future Oncol.,* 10(8), 1469-1486. doi: 10.2217/fon.14.19.

Moasser, M. M. (2014). Two dimensions in targeting HER2. *J. Clin. Oncol.,* 32(19), 2074-2077. doi: 10.1200/jco.2014.55.7652.

Pollock, N. I. and Grandis, J. R. (2014). HER2 as a Therapeutic Target in Head and Neck Squamous Cell Carcinoma. *Clin. Cancer Res.* doi: 10. 1158/1078-0432.ccr-14-1432.

Quesnelle, K. M. and Grandis, J. R. (2011). Dual kinase inhibition of EGFR and HER2 overcomes resistance to cetuximab in a novel in vivo model of acquired cetuximab resistance. *Clin. Cancer Res.,* 17(18), 5935-5944. doi: 10.1158/1078-0432.ccr-11-0370.

Romond, E. H., Perez, E. A., Bryant, J., Suman, V. J., Geyer, C. E., Jr., Davidson, N. E., ... Wolmark, N. (2005). Trastuzumab plus adjuvant chemotherapy for operable HER2-positive breast cancer. *N. Engl. J. Med.,* 353(16), 1673-1684. doi: 10.1056 /NEJMoa052122.

Sardari, Y., Pardis, S., Tadbir, A. A., Ashraf, M. J., Fattahi, M. J., Ebrahimi, H., ... Hamzavi, M. (2012). HER2/neu expression in head and neck squamous cell carcinoma patients is not significantly elevated. *Asian Pac. J. Cancer Prev.,* 13(6), 2891-2896.

Schechter, A. L., Stern, D. F., Vaidyanathan, L., Decker, S. J., Drebin, J. A., Greene, M. I., and Weinberg, R. A. (1984). The neu oncogene: an erb-B-related gene encoding a 185,000-Mr tumour antigen. *Nature,* 312(5994), 513-516.

Schrader, C., Boehm, A., Reiche, A., Dietz, A., Mozet, C., and Wichmann, G. (2012). Combined effects of lapatinib and cisplatin on colony formation of head and neck squamous cell carcinoma. *Anticancer Res.,* 32(8), 3191-3199.

Sequist, L. V., Yang, J. C., Yamamoto, N., O'Byrne, K., Hirsh, V., Mok, T., ... Schuler, M. (2013). Phase III study of afatinib or cisplatin plus pemetrexed in patients with metastatic lung adenocarcinoma with EGFR mutations. *J. Clin. Oncol.,* 31(27), 3327-3334. doi: 10.1200/jco.2012.44. 2806.

Shih, C., Padhy, L. C., Murray, M., and Weinberg, R. A. (1981). Transforming genes of carcinomas and neuroblastomas introduced into mouse fibroblasts. *Nature,* 290(5803), 261-264.

Slamon, D. J., Godolphin, W., Jones, L. A., Holt, J. A., Wong, S. G., Keith, D. E., ... et al. (1989). Studies of the HER-2/neu proto-oncogene in human breast and ovarian cancer. *Science,* 244(4905), 707-712.

Slamon, D. J., Leyland-Jones, B., Shak, S., Fuchs, H., Paton, V., Bajamonde, A., ... Norton, L. (2001). Use of chemotherapy plus a monoclonal antibody against HER2 for metastatic breast cancer that overexpresses HER2. *N. Engl. J. Med.,* 344(11), 783-792. doi: 10.1056/nejm200103153 441101.

Solca, F., Dahl, G., Zoephel, A., Bader, G., Sanderson, M., Klein, C., ... Adolf, G. R. (2012). Target binding properties and cellular activity of afatinib (BIBW 2992), an irreversible ErbB family blocker. *J. Pharmacol. Exp. Ther.,* 343(2), 342-350. doi: 10.1124 /jpet.112.197756.

Tzahar, E., Waterman, H., Chen, X., Levkowitz, G., Karunagaran, D., Lavi, S., ... Yarden, Y. (1996). A hierarchical network of interreceptor interactions determines signal transduction by Neu differentiation factor/neuregulin and epidermal growth factor. *Mol. Cell. Biol.,* 16(10), 5276-5287.

Ursini-Siegel, J., Schade, B., Cardiff, R. D., and Muller, W. J. (2007). Insights from transgenic mouse models of ERBB2-induced breast cancer. *Nat. Rev. Cancer,* 7(5), 389-397. doi: 10.1038/nrc2127.

Wei, Q., Sheng, L., Shui, Y., Hu, Q., Nordgren, H., and Carlsson, J. (2008). EGFR, HER2, and HER3 expression in laryngeal primary tumors and corresponding metastases. *Ann. Surg. Oncol.,* 15(4), 1193-1201. doi: 10. 1245/s10434-007-9771-3.

Williams, J. P., Kim, I., Ito, E., Shi, W., Yue, S., Siu, L. L., ... Liu, F. F. (2014). Pre-clinical characterization of Dacomitinib (PF-00299804), an irreversible pan-ErbB inhibitor, combined with ionizing radiation for head and neck squamous cell carcinoma. *PLoS One,* 9(5), e98557. doi: 10. 1371/journal.pone.0098557.

Wolff, A. C., Hammond, M. E., Schwartz, J. N., Hagerty, K. L., Allred, D. C., Cote, R. J., ... Hayes, D. F. (2007). American Society of Clinical Oncology/College of American Pathologists guideline recommendations for human epidermal growth factor receptor 2 testing in breast cancer. *Arch. Pathol. Lab. Med.,* 131(1), 18-43. doi: 10.1043/1543-2165(2007) 131[18:asocco]2.0.co;2.

Xia, W., Lau, Y. K., Zhang, H. Z., Liu, A. R., Li, L., Kiyokawa, N., ... Hung, M. C. (1997). Strong correlation between c-erbB-2 overexpression and overall survival of patients with oral squamous cell carcinoma. *Clin. Cancer Res.,* 3(1), 3-9.

Yan, M., Parker, B. A., Schwab, R., and Kurzrock, R. (2014). HER2 aberrations in cancer: implications for therapy. *Cancer Treat. Rev.,* 40(6), 770-780. doi: 10.1016/j.ctrv. 2014.02.008.

Yarden, Y. and Sliwkowski, M. X. (2001). Untangling the ErbB signalling network. *Nat. Rev. Mol. Cell Biol.,* 2(2), 127-137. doi: 10.1038/35052073.

In: Head and Neck Cancer
Editor: Madison R. Hall

ISBN: 978-1-63482-113-1

Chapter 4

Current Trends and Management in Head and Neck Cancers

***Arutha Kulasinghe*[1]*, Yenkai Lim*[1]*, Chris F. L. Perry*[2,3] *and Chamindie Punyadeera*[1*]**

[1]Queensland University of Technology, Institute of Health and Biomedical Innovations, Kelvin Grove, Australia

[2]Department of Otolaryngology, Princess Alexandra Hospital, Woolloongabba, Australia and the University of Queensland, the School of Medicine, Herston, Australia

Abstract

There is a general lack of public awareness on the daunting statistics of head and neck squamous cell carcinoma (HNSCC) when compared with other mainstay cancers such as breast and prostate cancers. HNSCC includes malignancies in five major anatomical sites, namely, oral cavity, oropharynx, nasopharynx, hypopharynx and larynx. HNSCC is diverse in nature both biologically and clinically. HNSCC is the 6th most common cancer globally with less than 50% survival beyond 5 years. Risk factors include smoking and alcohol consumption, betel nut chewing, wearing dentures, trauma to the gums and oral cavity as well as exposure to the human papillomavirus (HPV). HNSCC is more prevalent in men, however, the prevalence in women has been increasing due to changes in lifestyle over the last few decades. Whilst, smoking associated HNSCC is on the decline, HPV associated HNSCC is increasing. The therapy of choice for newly diagnosed patients consists of combined modality treatment of surgery, chemotherapy and radiotherapy. Despite this aggressive first line treatment, over 30% of HNSCC patients develop locoregional and distant metastasis and succumb to the disease. Early diagnostics are the key to early interventions at the disease stage which can improve patient outcomes. This chapter aims to outline HNSCC trends and statistics, research based prognostic and diagnostic tools, treatments and patient management.

[*] Correspondence: Associate Professor Chamindie Punyadeera; Institute of Health and Biomedical Innovations, Queensland University of Technology; 60 Musk Avenue, GPO Box 2434; Brisbane QLD 4001; Australia.

1. Head and Neck Squamous Cell Carcinoma

Head and neck squamous cell carcinoma (HNSCC) refers to cancer around the upper aerodigestive regions [1]. These regions include the oral cavity, nasal cavity, paranasal sinuses, pharynx and larynx [1, 2] (see Fig 1.). HNSCC originates from the mucosal lining in the head and neck region with squamous cell carcinoma as the most common histological variant, comprising 90% of all cancer types [3-5]. As the sixth most common cancer worldwide, HNSCC is responsible for 900,000 new cases and 300,000 deaths annually [1]. With poor prognosis, HNSCC patients have a five-year mortality rate of 40 to 50% [5-7]. Despite improvements in the locoregional control and reduced treatment-related morbidities, the five-year survival rates in HNSCC have not improved [8]. The lower 5-year survival rate is due to the late diagnosis of HNSCC (i.e. at stage II) and often associated with cervical lympnode metastasis [9]. In addition, it has also been reported that only 30% of HNSCC cases in the USA are diagnosed at an early clinical stage and two-thirds of patients present with advanced stage III or IV tumours [10]. The lack of early diagnostic methods are responsible for poor five-year survival rate [11].

Successful treatments in HNSCC patients rely on early detection and targeted therapy for each cancer subtype. However, currently most cases of HNSCC are detected when the patient has become symptomatic from the effects of the primary disease or when lymphatic metastases are palpable. Despite the obvious advantages of earlier diagnosis of HNSCC, no strategy is currently being implemented to effectively treat HNSCC patients at an earlier stage when the tumour burden is minimal (*i.e.* during neoplasia).

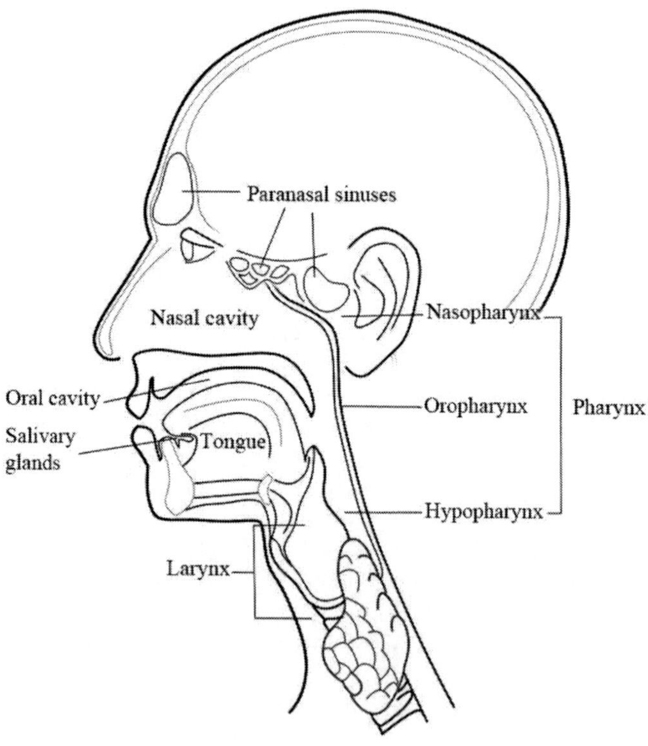

Figure 1. Anatomical sites where head and neck cancers arise.

Over the past five years, high incidence of HNSCC was reported in Southeast Asia, Central and Southeast Europe [1]. Increasing trends of HNSCC was also observed in Central, and Eastern Europe, Scandinavia, Canada, Japan and Australia [1]. In contrast, an overall decreasing trend was noted in India, Hong Kong, Brazil, USA and West Africa [1]. The majority of the people who develop HNSCC are in their sixth and seventh decades (93.3%) [12]. Men are at a 2-fold higher risk of developing HNSCC than women [13]. Tobacco & alcohol consumptions and Human papilloma virus (HPV) as well as genetic susceptibility (others include poor diet, betel nut chewing and mouth wash use) are major risk factors for developing HNSCC [1, 2, 14, 15]. Tobacco use has decreased over the past decade in high-income and upper middle-income countries due to the successful tobacco awareness campaigns [1]. However, there is an increasing trend of tobacco use in many developing countries, contributing to the increase prevalence of HNSCC [1]. As an example, oral cancers are higher in the Asian sub-continent [1]. In contrast, alcohol consumption is more popular in developed countries [1]. Overall, in the past five years, there has been no significant change in the rate of alcohol consumption worldwide [1]. Genetic predisposition also plays a major role in HNSCC development [1]. Patients suffering from Fanconi anemia, FAMMM, Bloom's syndrome, Xeroderma pigmentosum, Ataxia telangiectasia and Li-Fraumeni have 700 to 1000 fold risk of developing HNSCC compared to normal individuals [1]. These patients usually develop HNSCC at a younger age [1].

Currently, a slight decrease in the incidence of smoking associated HNSCC is documented [16]. Excessive tobacco and alcohol consumption remain important risk factors of HNSCC, however the global incidence of HPV-positive HNSCC (oropharyngeal squamous cell carcinoma, OPSCC) is on the rise. Over the past decade, there has been a rise of over 70% prevalence of HPV related oropharyngeal SCCs with the prevalence in Europe increasing at a faster rate than North America. In contrast to HPV-negative HNSCC, HPV-positive HNSCC targets young patients within the third and fourth decade due to high oral sex activities. As such, 89% of HPV-associated HNSCC are based within the oral cavity and oropharyngeal anatomical sites. Approximately 90% of HPV-related oropharyngeal cancers are due to HPV-16 subtype infections and most often found in the tonsils and base of tongue. It is estimated that tumours in the oropharynx are five times more likely to be HPV positive than those in the oral cavity, larynx or hypopharynx [17]. Locoregional control is also significantly better in HPV-positive OPSCC but the rate of distant metastasis increases after two years unlike in patients with HPV-negative tumours [18]. Furthermore metastases are more likely to occur significantly later in HPV-positive OPSCC compared to HPV-negative tumours, involving multiple organs, such as the skin, intra-abdominal lymph nodes and the brain [19]. However, the implication of HPV status on non-oropharyngeal sites on prognosis and distant metastases remains unclear. What is of interest is that, patients present with a more favourable prognosis. Patients tend to respond with better outcomes to combined modality chemoradiotherapy as well as stand-alone surgery. HPV status has been clinically relevant and played an important role in the treatment regimens of patients.

HPV-positive HNSCCs have genetic alterations that are direct result of HPV oncoproteins, E6 and E7, which inactivate the tumour suppressor gene products, p53 and Rb respectively. In HPV, the functional inactivation of p53 and pRB results in over expression of p16INK4A (p16); the inhibitor of cyclin-dependent kindases (CDK) in a negative feedback loop. Therefore p16 expression by immunohistochemistry (IHC) and/or in situ hybridization (ISH) for high risk HPV DNA has provided a routine clinical assay for rapid HPV detection screens in patients. p16 overexpression by IHC has become the surrogate screening marker for HPV positive HNSCC.

2. Epidemiology of Head and Neck Cancers

The rate of incidence of HNSCC is significantly higher in Southeast Asia and Eastern Europe compared to other regions due to geographic differences in ethnicity, culture and socioeconomics [18]. Table 1 summaries the global epidemiology of HNSCC per anatomical site.

Table 1. The summary of head and neck squamous cell carcinoma epidemiology worldwide based on the anatomical site of tumour origin [20]

Cancer location	Incidence (2010)		Mortality (2010)	
	Male	Female	Male	Female
Oral cavity and lip	170496	92524	83109	44545
Nasopharynx	57852	26589	35984	15609
Other pharynx	108588	28034	76458	19092
Larynx	129651	21026	70336	11556

The incidence of HNSCC in Australia rose from 2475 in 1982 to 3896 in 2009 (22% increase) [19]. However, the incidence rate has fallen from 19.3 per 100000 persons in 1982 to 16.8 per 100000 persons in 2009 due to an increase in life expectancy [21]. As of 2009, incidence of HNSCC in males were 73.8% while incidence of HNSCC in females was 26.2% [21]. In terms of mortality, the number of HNSCC deaths increased from 752 in 1998 to 944 in 2011 (11% increase) [21]. HNSCC survival rate improved via 6.4% across the 20th and 21st century [21]. Table 1.1 summaries the epidemiology of HNSCC in Australia for each anatomical site.

Table 1.1. The summary of head and neck squamous cell carcinoma epidemiology in Australia based on anatomical sites [21]

Cancer location	Incidence (2009)	Incidence rate (2009)	Mortality rates (1982-2011)	Survival rate (2006-2010)
Oral cavity	2037	8.8/100000 persons	1.5 deaths/100000 persons	75%
Pharynx	739	3.2/100000 persons	1.2 deaths/100000 persons	55.50%
Larynx	606	2.6/100000 persons	1.2 deaths/100000 persons	64.80%
Salivary glands	265	1.2/100000 persons	0.3 deaths/100000 persons	70.40%
Nasal cavity and paranasal sinus	166	0.8/100000 persons	0.2 deaths/100000 persons	60.30%

In the United Kingdom (UK), HNSCC accounts for less than 5% of all cancers [20]. There are more than 150 new HNSCC cases each year [22]. The HNSCC incidence rate in Thames and Oxford region are roughly around 8 per 100000 persons whilst in Wales and the North-western region have a higher incidence rate of 13 to 15 per 100000 persons [22]. The most common HNSCC in the UK are oral cavity and pharynx, in which the incidence rate of both cancer types have increased by 20% over the last three decades [22] (Table 1.2).

Table 1.2. The summary of head and neck squamous cell carcinoma epidemiology in United Kingdom based on anatomical sites [22]

Cancer location	Incidence (2010)		
	Cases	Male	Female
Oral cavity	4329	62%	38%
Oropharynx	1456	73%	27%
Other	754	74%	26%

HNSCC is the 8th most common cancer in the United States [21]. Similar to the United Kingdom, HNSCC accounts for 3 to 5% of all cancers in the United States [22]. In 2014, it is estimated that there will be 55070 new HNSCC cases with 12000 deaths [22]. Compared with the estimated figure of 47500 HNSCC cases in 2008, the incidence rate decreased due to increased population and life expectancy [22] (see Table 1.3).

Table 1.3. The summary of head and neck squamous cell carcinoma epidemiology in United States based on anatomical sites [24]

Cancer location	Incidence (1973-2006)	Survival rate (2002-2006)
Oral cavity	19221	62.9%
Nasopharynx	4745	62.3%
Oropharynx	2014	42.2%
Larynx	28348	66.8%

HNSCC is a major problem in India, it accounts for 30 to 40% of all cancer [23][24]. There are over 200000 new cases of HNSCC in India each year [25-26]. It is the sixth most common cause of death in males and seventh in females [25-26]. On a global scale, India contributes 31% to pharyngeal cancers and 18% to laryngeal cancers every year [25-26]. Bhopal alone, has the world's highest rate of HNSCC incidence in the oral cavity in males [25-26]. However, a slow decreasing trend in incidence can be observed in all anatomical sites in general except for the oral cavity [25-26]. This is due to the etiological factor of betel quid abuse [25-26]. In India, HNSCC has a clear predilection towards males at 79% of the total HNSCC cases [25-26] (see Figure 2). Unfortunately, no statistical data is available from India (Figure 2).

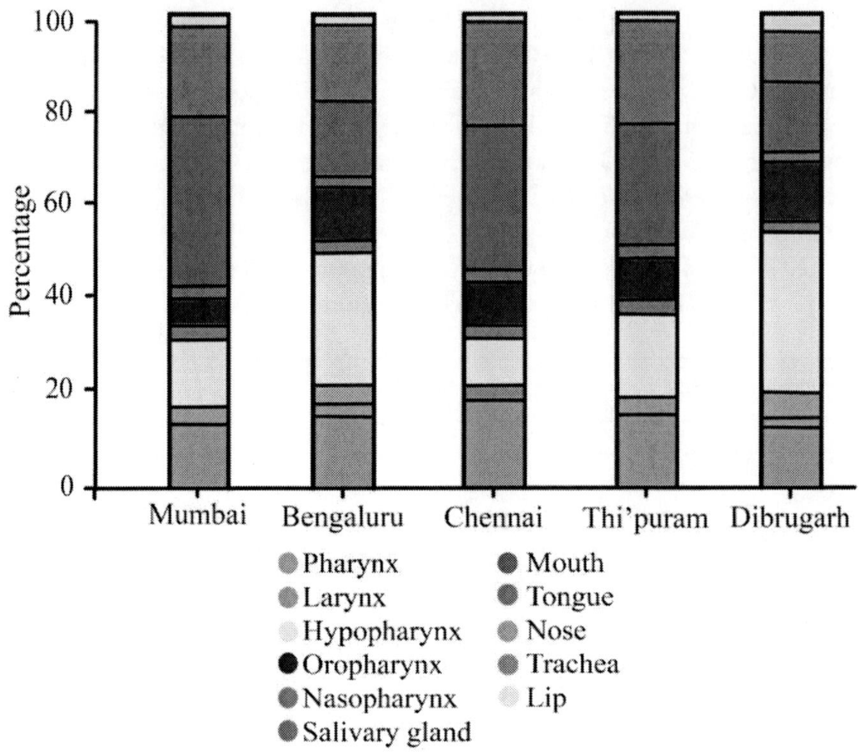

Figure 2. The summary of head and neck squamous cell carcinoma epidemiology in males in India (2004-2006) based on anatomical sites [25].

3. Pathogenesis of Head and Neck Cancers

The pathogenesis of HNSCC is considered as a multistep process which begins with the accumulation of genetic alterations leading to aberrant protein expression facilitating tumour growth and progression. HNSCC arises due to a series of molecular alterations giving rise from dysplasia to carcinoma in situ, and finally invasive carcinoma. There are genetic and epigenetic alterations in pre-cancerous cells that contribute to transformation of these cells into malignant forms. The factors that govern the transformation of pre-cancer cells into malignant transformations include accumulation of genetic alterations as well as tumour microenvironment which enables tumour progression. Genetic and epigenetic changes (DNA methylation and miRNA over or under expression as well as aberent histone modifications) lead to protein changes affecting tumour initiation and progression.

Epigenetic and genetic alterations differ between HPV-positive and HPV-negative HNSCCs. Examples of altered pathways in HNSCC include p53, epidermal growth factor receptor (EGFR), signal transducer and activator of transcription 3 (STAT3) and vascular endothelial growth factor receptor (VEGFR).

(i) p53 Pathway

TP53 is a well-known frequently mutated HNSCC gene. It is a tumour suppressor gene that is a transcription factor and regulates many downstream gene targets in response to cellular stress. In HNSCC, it has been estimated that between 46-73% of cases have this p53 mutation [25-27]. As an example, in HPV-negative tumours, the p53 gene is one of the most commonly mutated genes with mutations detected in over 50% of HNSCC malignancies. In contrast, p53 is wild-type in HPV-positive HNSCC tumours. TP53 is made up of 393 amino acids and 4 domains including a highly conserved region which play important roles in cellular mechanisms including responses to DNA damage and oncogenic stressors [27].

In normal cells, p53 is activated via stress signals such as DNA-double strand break or aberrant growth signals and activates the transcription of genes necessary for apoptosis and the inhibition of cell cycle progression. When DNA damage and/or a multitude of stress signals, p53 can induce expression of Bax leading to apoptosis. Due to either double stranded DNA break or aberrant growth signal activation, p53 increases the expression of p21 and p21 inhibits cyclin-dependent kinases (CDKs) leading to the inhibition of cell cycle progression from the G1 phase to the S phase [28]. Inactivation of the tumour suppressor p53 on chromosome 17q13 leads to aberent cell growth control and renders cells unable to respond to stress or DNA damage. Moreover, other genes in the p53 pathway are often mutated or dysregulated causing dysfunction of the p53 pathway. As an example, silencing of Ataxia telangiectasia mutated (ATM, is a kinase) is a mechanism of loss-of-function of p53 [29]. p14arf lies upstream of p53 and binds the p53 inhibitor HDM2 in order to activate p53. Mutations in ARF locus expression is a common molecular event in the pathogenesis of HNSCC.

(ii) Epidermal Growth Factor Receptor Pathway

Epidermal Growth Factor Receptor Pathway (EGFR) is a member of the HER/erb B family of tyrosine kinase receptors that is highly expressed in epithelial cells. EGFR mediates multiple signalling pathways that control, proliferation, invasion, migration, survival and angiogenesis. EGFR pathway is upstream of phosphoinositol-3-kinase (PI3K), Akt as well as the mitogen activated protein kinase pathways (MAPK, stimulated through the Ras/Raf pathway). EGFR (ErbB-1 or HER1) is a tyrosine kinase receptor that is highly expressed in epithelial cells. Due to EGFR gene amplifications and transcriptional activations in HNSCC, EGFR is ubiquitously expressed in HNSCC [30, 31]. EGFR pathway is activated by autocrine growth factors such as TGFalpha, amphiregulin as well as EGF. When EGF binds to EGFR, EGFR dimerizes, autophosphorylation occurs and downstream signalling is activated. Besides the over expression of EGFR, a mutant form of EGFR known as EGFRvIII, which is characterized by a deletion mutation in exons 2–7 give rise to a truncated ligand binding domain, rendering it constitutively active [32]. In a clinical setting, therapeutics targeting EGFR have been used for HNSCC. Cetuximab, which is a chimeric murine/human monocolonal antibody which is used against EGFR has been used in locally advanced stage and metastatic patients with improved survival in these patients over standard therapies [27].

(iii) Signal Transducers and Activators of Transcription Pathway

STAT-3 is a transcriptional factor downstream of EGFR pathway and facilitates in tumourigenesis.

Activation of STAT-3 besides EGFR pathway includes the activation of src kinases as well as the interleukin-6 (IL-6)/gp130 receptor pathway through janus kinase (JAK) mediated phosphorylation [16]. STAT3 activation leads to transcriptional activation of genes that control cell cycle progression, apoptosis and angiogenesis including Cyclin D1, Bcl-XL and VEGF.

(iv) Vascular Endothelial Growth Factor and Receptor Pathway

In numerous tumour types including HNSCC, STAT3 induces the expression of VEGF. VEGF binds to VEGFR which are found on endothelial cells that leads to the initiation of angiogenesis. The binding of VEGF to its receptor on endothelial cells results in endothelial proliferation, migration and an increase in the permeability of the vasculature. Lymphatic endothelial cells also show an increase in the expression of endothelial specific adhesion molecule (esam1), VEGFR-3, transforming growth factors beta 2 (TGF β2) and platelet derived growth factor beta (PDGF-β2) [33]. In HNSCC patients expressing high levels of VEGF and VEGF receptor, it has been shown to correlate to poor patient outcomes and worse survival as a result of higher tumour proliferative rates [34].

(v) Transforming Growth Factor-β (TGF-β) / Ras Pathway

TGF-β plays an important role in cell differentiation, regeneration and regulatory functions of the immune system. TGF-β receptors are from the family of serine/threonine kinase receptors.

The pathways that Ras signal transduction regulate include proliferation, migration, differentiation, cell adhesion, apoptosis as well as the regulation of cytoskeletal composition [34]. Dysregulation of Ras activation has been associated with malignancy. Ras overexpression is common in HNSCC whereas Ras mutations are rare [35]. Studies suggest that Ras may play a role in tumour initiation whereas TGF-β appears to present with tumour progression effects at a later stage.

4. Current Diagnostic Strategies for Head and Neck Cancers

Despite the rapid advancements in cancer diagnostics over the past four decades, there has been marginal improvements in the survival of HNSCC patients [36]. This is further complicated by the heterogeneity of HNSCC and variations in tissues of origin. These can range from mucosal epithelia in the oral cavity, pharynx and larynx. Therefore, HNCs are considered to be a heterogeneous disease representing a plethora of histology and differentiation patterns [37].

For the last forty to fifty years the evolution of HNC treatments has been based on outcome measures for the differing treatment options available. Tumours are first pigeon-holed into different categories containing similar tumours using the Tumour, Nodal and distant Metastatic (TNM) classifications of size on presentation as an indicator of aggressiveness and how advanced and overwhelming a cancer has become. The size and extent of a tumour on presentation is assessed clinically and radiologically using the TNM staging system. Historically two systems were in use – the UICC 1 (Union for International

Cancer Control) and the AJCC 2 (American Joint Committee on Cancer). These classifications have evolved over time to more accurately reflect prognosis, and are now similar/interchangeable. The T classification goes from levels one to four with increasing size indicated by an increased T number. T1 is a small tumour. Currently a T4a tumour is very large but possibly still curable, while a T4b lesion is generally so advanced and destructive locally that the chance of cure is quite small. Similarly an N1 is small – a single node less than 3cm in size, whereas an N3 is large (> 6 cm), and often fixed by invading surrounding structures with consequent decreased survival. The N2 nodal metastases take into account bigger nodes (3-6 cm), more than one node and bilaterality of nodes which all indicate worsening prognosis by adding 'a', 'b' and 'c' subsets (N2a, N2b, N2c). By looking at the survivals by T stage of various treatment modalities, real advances have finally been made over the last twenty five years, bearing in mind that radiotherapy has been available for only about one hundred years and only very small cancers are curable surgically before the last fifty years or so. Good reconstructive flaps have been available for about thirty to forty years and now microvascular free flaps are almost the norm in reconstruction.

It has been standard of care for some time now that the large centres have multidisciplinary clinics and teams (MDT) to assess a patients' TNM stage and then suggest the ideal modality of therapy, bearing in mind all the factors involved in actually determining what is the best treatment for that individual patient is. The patients' age, immune-competence, their general health and their wishes all play a part in determining their best treatment option. Tumour factors include the TNM staging, the differentiation, and the presence of viral markers. Local expertise factors come in to play, as well as the availability of drugs and treatment, including expertise of the surgeon and radiation oncologist. What radiotherapy machines are available and whether there is local expertise in the more technically challenging Intensity Modulated Radiotherapy (IMRT) also plays a part. Generally in OECD countries funding should be adequate, but there is a misdistribution of health funding across many OECD countries [38]. The treatment options for most patients in developing countries are limited and this effects survival chances for the patient [39].

Upon presentation to the clinic, patients will be physically and visually examined by the clinicians. These inspections can be carried out by the use of a spatula and as such they are able to reach areas that are hidden within the head and neck regions, palpitation of lymph nodes around the neck area. For other areas of the head and neck which are difficult to see, clinicians may use various equipments. These include nasoendoscopy, laryngoscopy and tissue biopsy (sampling). Nasendoscopy is an examination of the nose or throat using a flexible fibre optic cable which has a light and camera attached to one end. It is a form of an endoscope. A numbing agent or local anaesthetic is sprayed within the area to numb and as such there is minimal pain to the patients when the nasoendoscope is passed through. The nasendoscopy allows the clinician to look into the patients nasal cavity, nasopharynx, oropharynx and larynx easily and can be viewed in real-time. The examination is termed by various names depending on the area of examination, for example, if the larynx is viewed; laryngoscopy, pharynx; pharyngoscopy. When these areas are combined during a clinical examination, it is referred to as a panendoscopy [40].

Medical imaging is another means of diagnosing HNSCC and includes techniques such as ultrasound, x-rays, computed tomography (CT/CAT) scan, Magnetic resonance imaging (MRI) or Positron emission tomography (PET) scan. Ultrasound scans use sound waves to create an image of the internal organs. X-rays of the head and neck regions are quick and painless. Chest x-rays may be done for patients with mouth or pharyngeal cancers to assess whether the cancer have spread to the lungs. X rays of facial bones may also be done for signs of spreading of the cancer. CT scans are able to create three-dimensional images of the body with an x-ray machine. This allows for cross sectional views showing abnormalities in the body and possible tumours. The dimensions of the tumours may be measured using a CT scan. This allows the radiologist to stage the patient according to tumour size, nodal spread and metastasis, commonly called TNM. A MRI scan uses magnets and magnetic fields to produce detailed images of the body, notably soft tissue in the head and neck region such as the tongue and tonsils. A contrast dye may be given to the patient prior to the scan to produce better imaging. PET scans use a small amount of radioactive dye, which is taken up by cells with the highest metabolic turn around, in particular, tumour cells. Due to the biology of cancer cells and their tendency to use energy actively, it absorbs more of the radioactive dye and this shows up on imaging.

When the tumours are visible, then a biopsy is taken from the suspicious anatomical site for routine histopathological examinations by a pathologist. The biopsy is the 'gold standard' for a definitive diagnosis. The pathologist is specialized in the analysis and interpretation of cells, tissues and organs to diagnose disease. A common type of biopsy in head and neck cancer is a fine needle aspiration (FNA). During a FNA, cells are taken up from a tissue by a thin needle inserted directly into the tumour or lymph node. The cells are then examined under a microscope to determine whether there are abnormal/ cancer cells, termed a cytologic examination. Further molecular testing on a tumour sample may be recommended by a consulting doctor for identification of genes and proteins. These results would allow the doctor to treat a patient based on the clinical confirmatory diagnosis. Currently, there is no consensus on the optimal way to identify HPV-positive HNSCC. The different methods include the detection of p16 protein expression using IHC as well as HPV-related genetic material using polymerase chain reaction (PCR) and ISH in tumour biopsy samples. In addition, the presence of HPV-specific antibodies in serum has also been associated with increased risk of developing OPSCC [41].

p16 Immunohistochemistry

During immortalisation of host cells, the E7 protein of High risk (HR-HPV-16) binds to Rb, resulting in the compensatory over-expression of the tumour suppressor gene p16 in HPV-infected tumour cells [42]. The IHC analysis of p16INK4A in HNSCC tumour biopsies has been shown to serve as a surrogate marker to identify HPV infection in histologic preparations from HNSCCs [43]. However, in a pooled analysis of 496 patients with OPSCC from different studies utilizing DNA-based HPV testing, 5% of cases were p16INK4A positive/HPV negative and 8% were p16INK4A negative/HPV positive [44]. Another study has shown that p16INK4A is also over-expressed in a subset of HNSCC lacking HPV DNA, is close to 14% of tumours that were p16 positive were negative by HPV-specific ISH and PCR [45]. Strikingly, Hoffmann et al. reported that no over-expression of p16INK4A was observed in 3/14 (21.4%) patients who were positive for HPV DNA and mRNA [46]. Furthermore, Harris et al. demonstrated an over-expression of p16 in young patients with oral tongue SCC without evidence of HPV infections [47-49]. Liang et al also showed that OPSCC patients who were p16 positive and seronegative for HPV antibodies had significantly increased hazard of all causes of death [48]. These data support the notion that p16 over expression alone is not sufficient to accurately identify HPV infection in HNSCC. However, p16 IHC has been shown to be a suitable test for risk stratifying patients with OPSCC as p16 positivity in tumour correlates with better survival [49]. p16 IHC has been adopted as the single test of choice for many medical practitioners due to the fact that it has been extensively studied, cost effective with clear staining interpretation guidelines [49]. Direct identification of HPV using DNA and RNA-based methods will still be required for clinically relevant infection and may replace p16 IHC or used in conjunction with it [49].

Premalignant lesions/precancerous lesions demonstrate histological changes consistent with an increased risk of progression to squamous cell carcinoma. The changes may include hyperplasia and dysplasia. Leukoplakia is a term used to describe a white patch or plaque which cannot be rubbed off. The prevalence in the US is almost 3%, most commonly found in patients ranging 50-70 years. Tobacco use is consistently found in this patient population. Other reasons which may lead to white patches include dental trauma and chronic irritation of the area [34]. Erythroplakia is characteristically red and presents with a velvet-like presentation and clear borders. This is the most common presentation of early HNSCC with approximately half of erythroplakic lesions possibly harbouring invasive HNSCC. These lesions do not subside.

(i) Squamous Dysplasia

Squamous dysplasia occurs when certain architectural features appear such as 'drop-shaped' rete ridges, keratin pearly, irregularities in the epithelial stratification, abnormal superficial mitosis and loss of cellular polarity. There are certain criteria involved in the grading of dysplasia such as variations in the nucleus size, the cellular morphology, shape, nuclear to cytoplasmic ratios, atypical mitotic figures as well as dyskeratosis [34].

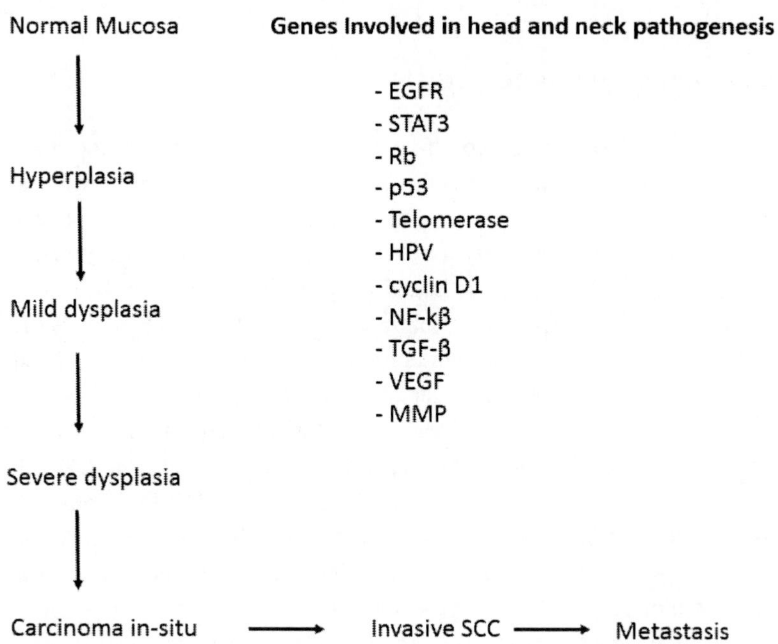

Figure 3. The development of head and neck cancers from premalignant lesions.

(ii) Carcinoma in-Situ

Carcinoma in-situ (CIS) presents a malignant transformation process, however invasion has not taken place. The characteristic trait of malignancy is that of invasion which is easily determined by cytologically abnormal squamous cells showing perineural or vascular infiltration. The presentation of an invasive HNSCC include atypical squamous cells with atypical nuclei, increased nucleus to cytoplasmic ratio, atypical mitotic figures, basement membrane invasion and an inflammatory response [34]. Moreover, the invasive cells tend to become more mesenchymal-like reflecting their aggressive nature [36].

5. Molecular Techniques to Determine Distant Metastasis in Head and Neck Cancers

The presence of metastatic disease in the cervical lymph nodes of HNC patients significantly affects the resulting therapy and prognosis for the patients. Accurate staging of the locoregional metastasis is important [50]. However, current clinically available diagnostic tools (CT scans, MRI and PET scans) do not allow for the detection of micrometastasis. Micrometastatic deposits (smaller than 5mm) cannot be detected with the current imaging techniques[51]. An invasive approach would be an ultrasound guided fine-needle aspiration. Cytology, as a tool also has limitations in its sensitivity. These limitations in staging have resulted in elective treatment of the neck, generally by neck dissection in surgically treated patients. Whilst this is effective, it does come with morbidity risks [52]. Molecular tests could allow for better diagnostics by the detection of micrometastasis and the identification of mutations in the circulating cancer cells which has led to their entry into the lymphovasculature [36, 53].

5.1. The Detection of Micrometastasis

A strategy that has been employed for the detection of micrometastasis is that of circulating tumour cells (CTCs) in the peripheral blood of HNC patients by the expression of epithelial cancer specific markers [54]. Currently, there are multiple approaches to isolate and characterize these cells, however, only one U.S. Food and Drug Administration (FDA) approved technology. This technology is based on positive immunomagnetic enrichment of cells using expression of the epithelial cell adhesion molecule (EpCAM). In metastatic prostate, breast and colon cancer, the enumeration of CTCs has been correlated to survival and disease outcomes [54]. However, larger studies are required in HNCs to evaluate the clinical utility of CTCs in patient management. A clinical trial has begun in France at the University Hospital Montpellier where they aim to utilize the CellSearch®, EPISPOT and flow cytometer to detect and characterize viable CTCs in HNSCC patients [55]. More importantly, as a result of a large scaled pooled analysis in breast cancer, distant metastases have been included in the cancer staging. cM0(i+) indicating that no clinical or radiographic evidence of distant metastases, but "deposits of molecularly or microscopically detected tumour cells in circulating bloods, bone marrow or other non-regional nodal tissue [56]. Numerous isolation devices are currently under review; incorporating positive/negative selection techniques, size based isolation, microfluidic approaches to capture the largest possible population of CTCs in a background of normal blood cells. Other avenues that researchers are looking into implement are circulating tumour DNA (ctDNA) which research groups have been able to detect in early and late stages of malignancies, however the use of ctDNA over CTCs is currently under vigorous debate [57]. In a recent study by Bettegowda et al., 2014, demonstrated that ctDNA was detectable in the absence of CTCs suggesting that ctDNA and CTCs were separate entities and that ctDNA is a sensitive and specific biomarker across numerous cancer types including pancreatic, ovarian, bladder, breast and head and neck [58]. Epithelial-mesenchymal transition (EMT) is a complex process which leads to increase motility and cell dedifferentiation and is thought to be one of the key transitions that cells undergo in order to intravasate into the vasculature. CTCs are thought to arise from these epithelial cells in the primary tissue which lose their epithelial antigens, gain migratory and invasive capabilities causing disruptions to the basements and extracellular matrix, expressing markers of the EMT transition and presenting with a mesenchymal phenotype [36]. In HNSCC cells, it has been shown that EGFR, neurothropin receptor B (TrkB) and inflammatory cytokines (interleukin-1β) are involved in EMT [59]. The reverse process of mesenchymal-epithelial transition (MET), where mesenchymal cells re-gain their epithelial phenotype is thought to allow CTCs to seed at distant sites such as the lungs, liver and bone for HNSCC. It has been suggested that CTCs presenting with high EMT/MET plasticity tend to be the most aggressive [60].

6. Biomarkers for Head and Neck Cancers

The definition of a biomarker varies and currently there is no one definition that encompasses all aspects of biomarker applications. A biomarker, or biological marker as termed by the World Health Organisation (WHO) is defined as "any substance, structure, or process that can be measured in the body or its products and influence or predict the incidence of outcome or disease [61]."

According to the National Cancer Institute's (NCI) Early Detection Research Network (EDRN) define biomarkers as cellular, biochemical, molecular, or genetic alterations by which a normal, abnormal, or simply biologic process can be recognized or monitored [62].

A broader definition includes the effects of treatment, interventions and the influences of environmental exposure. This definition describes the usefulness of biomarkers for diagnostic purposes by detecting the presence of pathogenic processes or the absence of normal biological processes in disease. A biomarker may be a molecule that is secreted during malignancy itself, or it can be a specific response of the body to the presence of cancer [63].

The biomarkers can be for (a) diagnostic (commonly used in people with signs and symptoms to aid in assessing whether they have a condition); (b) screening (used in asymptomatic people to detect a disease or condition at an early stage) and (c) prognostic (used in subjects diagnosed with a condition to predict subsequent outcomes). The potential for earlier diagnosis compared to current methodology is what makes biomarkers a promising research avenue. The clinical benefits of early diagnostics are great and more importantly presymptomatic screening becomes vital due to an aging and a growing world population.

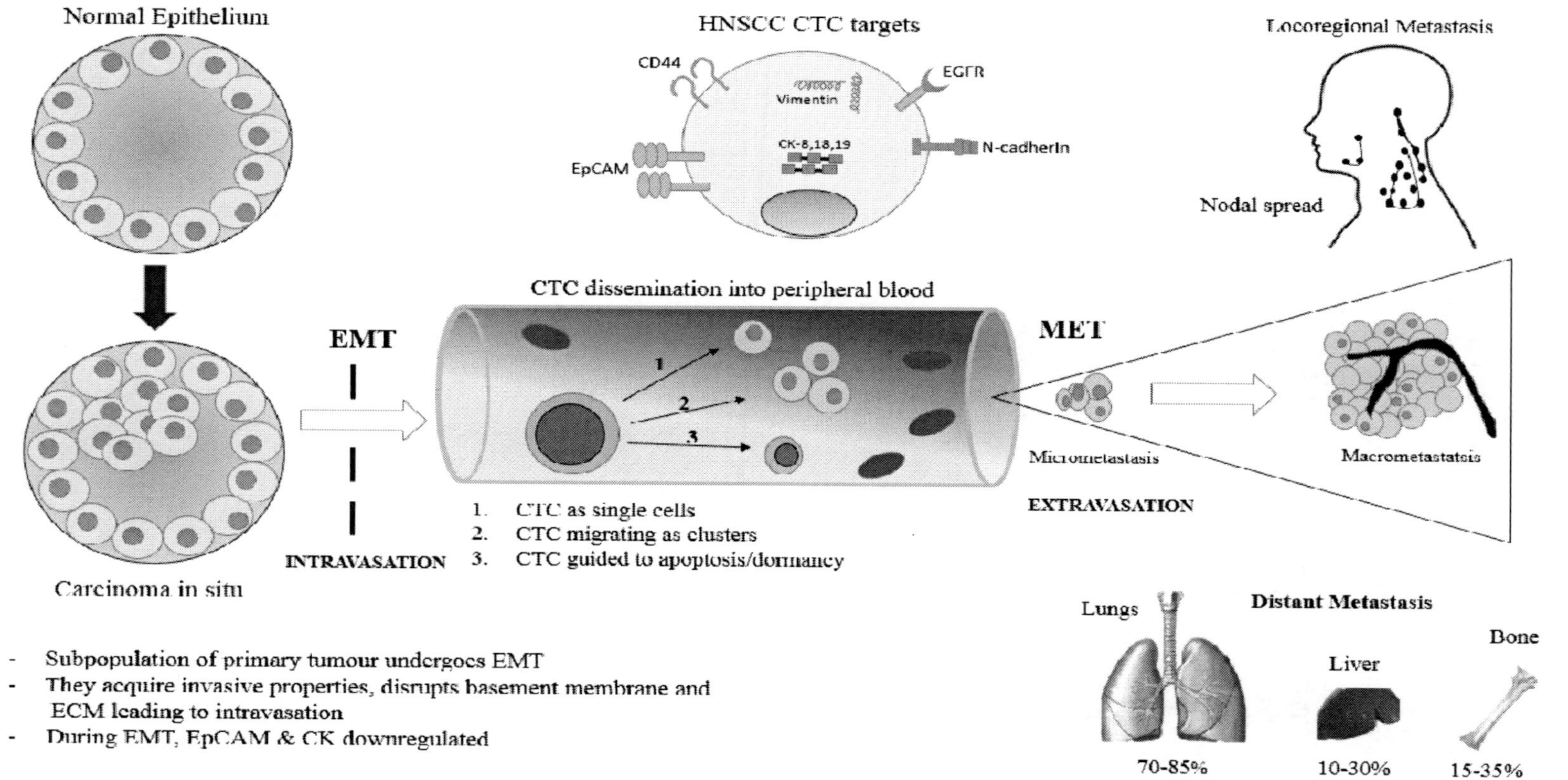

Figure 4. A subpopulation of the primary tumour that undergoes EMT and acquires invasive properties leading to intravasation into circulation. CTCs may be guided to apoptosis, some may survive and either circulate as singlet/doublets or clusters of cells. CTCs undergoing MET can lead to proliferation, angiogenesis and metastases (locoregional and/or distant). CTC: Circulating tumour cell; CK: Cytokeratin; CD44: Cell surface glycoprotein; EpCAM: Epithelial cell adhesion molecule; EGFR: Epidermal growth factor receptor; EMT: Epithelial-mesenchymal transition; MET: Mesenchymal-epithelial transition; ECM: Extra cellular matrix.

The ability for the early detection of disease is in its infancy provides clinicians with more treatment options as well as additional time to make more informed decisions and ultimately better patient outcomes and stratifications. The most relevant biological alterations in HNCs by frequency are FGFR3 (19%).

6.1. Biomarker Development

It is important to question as to why a large number of biomarker discoveries have not made it into the clinic. There are a large number of biomarker studies undertaken in the field of HNC investigating various body fluids as well as biomolecules ranging from proteins and their modifications, RNA, miRNA and DNA methylation [64]. One way to address this issue is to look into the requirements for biomarker development paying more attention to the study design. It is highly unlikely that a single marker would be a biomolecule that can differentiate between healthy and HNC patients due to disease heterogeneity. As an example, consider a biomarker with high sensitivity and low specificity. In this case this biomarker will identify people with the disease but fails to identify people who do not have the disease. This would mean that there is unnecessary healthcare costs added to the healthcare system and people who are free of disease may be targeted for treatments. Clearly, a biomarker should present good specificity and sensitivity.

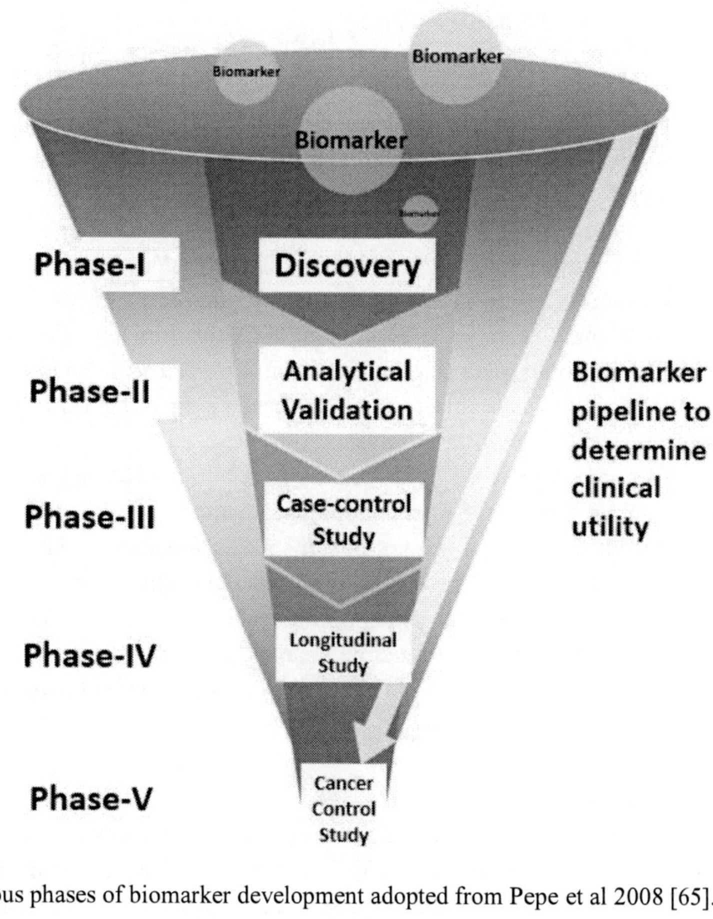

Figure 5. Various phases of biomarker development adopted from Pepe et al 2008 [65].

The key aspects of the clinical study design for each of the phases have been extensively discussed [65], which has generated ideas and many interesting thoughts on the clinical relevance and clinical translational of biomarkers. Pepe and colleagues proposed a prospective-specimen collection, retrospective-blinded-evaluation (PRoBE) design in which biologic specimens are collected prospectively from a cohort that represents the target population of interest for clinical application of the biomarker. Further, NCI's Early Detection Research Network (EDRN) has developed and implemented systematic, comprehensive guidelines to develop, evaluate, and validate biomarkers. This five-phase approach clearly defines the steps that should be adhered prior to the transition of biomarker(s) into a clinical setting. Phase 1 is called the validation phase and includes a feasibility study to identify potential candidate biomarkers. In Phase 2, the strategy would be to develop biomarkers that have higher differentiated capacity to distinguish between cases with HNSCC and controls without the disease. Phase 3 is designed to determine the capacity of biomarker(s) or panels to detect pre-clinical disease. Repositories of longitudinally collected clinical specimens from research cohorts are used. Phase 4 is designed as prospective screening study. Phase 5 is a large-scale population based study that evaluate the role of the biomarker(s) or panels for detection of HNSCC as well as the overall impact of screening the general population. Future biomarker development studies should follow this basic 5 steps pathway to succeed.

6.2. Biomarker Analysis in Body Fluids

Depending on the location of the tumour, one may not be able to access and swab the tumour bed. As an example, if the tumour is in the vocal cord area, it is difficult to take a biopsy without damaging the vocal cords. In such a setting, the use of human saliva may show unique advantages over the use of exfoliated cells. We and others have shown that one is able to detect early tumour activities in body fluids that drain from the organ that is affected by the tumour. As an example, the use of saliva to detect oral and oropharynx cancers is possible because the cancer-specific biomolecules are secreted in to saliva and by collecting and analysing the saliva, one is able to detect tumour activities [66-72]. We have shown in a recent publication that we could analyse HNSCC-specific miRNAs in saliva collected from HNSCC patients and we were also able to validate these findings also using the publically available data from The Cancer Genome Analysis [70].

Human saliva has come to the fore front recently as an alternative diagnostic medium for detecting oral and systemic diseases. Saliva is a multi-constituent oral bio-fluid which has the potential for use in the surveillance of general health and disease states. The National Cancer Institute in the USA has identified saliva as an important cancer biomarker fluid. Saliva can be used as a biological fluid as it has proteins, nucleic acids, electrolytes and hormones originating from a number of local and systemic sources. Moreover, it has been shown that saliva contains 30% of biomolecules found in blood. Listed below are some of the biomarkers found in body fluids.

(i) Microsatellite Instability

Microsatellite regions are genomic 1–5 bp tandem repeats, normally noncoding, and the CA 2 bp repeat is the most common form [73]. These regions may cause instability due to replication errors caused by DNA polymerase and is referred to as microsatellite instability

(MSI). Instability frequency is related to the repeat unit length and overall size of the short tandem repeat (STR), affecting the probability of error during DNA replication [74]. These replication errors can lead to tumourigenesis by activating oncogenes and silencing tumour suppressor genes. Two studies have identified MSI of D3S1611 in HNSCC markers with 13.5% and 40% [75, 76]. In contrast, a lack of MSI in HNSCC was reported by other studies [76, 77]. MSI studies showed lack of uniformity of the study methods, choice and number of markers. To date, no standard approach for the study of MSI has been developed for the early detection of HNSCC.

(ii) DNA Methylation

DNA methylation is an earlier tumorigenicity event in eukaryotes [78]. This process involves the attachment of a methyl group to the fifth carbon around the cytosine ring [79]. This formation creates an extension on the overall DNA alpha-helical structure [80]. Such extension hinders the binding of the transcription factor during DNA replication process, resulting suppressed expression of the involved genes [80]. In addition, transcription repressors have a predilection toward methylated promoters, this process further instigate the inactivation of the genes [80]. In a case where the involved genes function as tumour suppressor, it encourages the formation of neoplasm as the cells lose the ability to control cell-growth [4, 79, 80]. As such, DNA methylation of tumour suppressor genes are excellent biomarker(s) for the early detection of cancer [78]. Furthermore, researches have shown that alcohol and tobacco consumption have a strong correlation with the methylation level of tumour suppressor genes, indicating the use of these genes in large population based screening studies in high-risk individuals [78]. Numerous HNSCC biomarkers have been detected from the cancer secretome in saliva over the past decade [81-85]. These biomarkers show promising results when screening for HNSCC. In addition, certain biomarkers are able to determine the severity of the disease [5]. Some of the more popular HNSCC biomarkers in the field include Ras Association Domain Family 1 Isoform A (RASSF1a), Cyclin-dependent Kinase Inhibitor 2A (p16INK4a), Death-associated Protein Kinase 1 (DAPK1) and Methylguanine-DNA Methyltransferase (MGMT) [81-83, 85].

The method of choice to investigate the methylation status of a gene is though DNA bisulfite conversion, introduced by Formmer et al. in 1992 [79]. This method utilises sodium bisulfite ($NaHSO_3$) to actively induce oxidative deamination under the right conditions [79]. The reaction converts cytosine to uracil via replacing the amine group on the forth carbon with an oxide [79]. However, a methylated cytosine is significantly less susceptible to the reaction, holding the reaction backward by two order of magnitude . With two different primer sets (methylated-specific and unmethylated-specific) running in the same set of PCR [86 condition (methylation-specific PCR), the methylation status of a gene can be determine via quantifying the band intensity of an electrophoresis gel [87]. Other advanced DNA methylation analysis assays include mass spectrometry, multiplex-PCR and pyrosequencing [88].]

While DNA methylation status controls the expression level of a gene, miRNAs play an important role in post-transcriptional regulation [70]. miRNAs are small non-coding RNAs (approximately 22 nucleotides long) that function by targeting specific mRNA moieties for translational repression or degradation thereby regulating several biological process including cell proliferation, migration, invasion, survival and metastasis [70]. It is known that miRNAs are responsible for 67% of the gene expression in mammalian cells [70]. Currently, there are

1872 successfully identified human miRNA precursors, contributing to 2578 mature miRNAs [70]. miRNAs can be found within the intergenic, intronic or exonic regions in both protein-coding or non-protein-coding genes, together they constitute 3-5% of predicted genes in the human genome [70]. Many miRNAs have been identified in regions that are related to cancer causation [70]. These regions are usually responsible in cell proliferation, differentiation, apoptosis and cell cycle regulation [70]. As a result, many researchers believe that miRNAs may play a significant role in cancer outset, development and/or metastasis [70].

Table 2. The prominent DNA methylation biomarkers in saliva that have been associated with the development of head and neck cancers over the past five-years

Gene	Function	Reference
CCNA1	Cell cycle regulator	[5]
DAPK1	Programmed cell death	[5]
DCC	Receptor for nectrin required for axon guidance	[5]
EDNRB	G protein-coupled receptor	[5]
ERCC1	Nuclear hormone receptor	[5]
HOXA9	Promotes mammary epithelial cell growth and survival	[85]
KIF1A	Protein kinase involved in apoptosis and DNA damage response	[5]
MED-15	RNA polymerase II regulator	[89]
MGMT	DNA mismatch repair system	[5]
MINT-31	Calcium channel regulator	[5]
NID2	Cell adhesion	[85]
$p16^{INK2a}$	Receptor of sonic hedgehog	[5]
RASSF1a	Induce growth inhibition along the RAS-activated signalling pathway	[90]
TIMP3	T-cell antigen receptor, recognition of foreign antigens	[5]
PAX1	Transcription factor for chordate development	[91]
TCF21	Inhibitor of the matrix metalloproteinase	[7]

miRNAs in HNSCC have been extensively studied over the years, multiple miRNAs dysregulation were found in HNSCC cell lines that are specific to various anatomical sites, indicating the potential clinical utility as early diagnostic biomarkers [70]. Most HNSCC miRNA biomarker studies are carried out via miRNA PCR array assays to determine the the miRNA expression levels in HNSCC tumour cells compared to adjacent healthy cells [70]. According to literature, commonly up-regulated miRNA in HNSCC tumours include miR-363, miR-497, miR-33, miR-21, miR-31, miR-195star, miR-150, miR-146b-5p, miR-15a, miR-20b and miR-146a while commonly down-regulated miRNAs in HNSCC include miR-155, miR-181a, miR-181b, miR-29a, miR-218, miR-222, miR-221, miR-143-5p, miR-375 and miR-133a [70]. In recent publications, miR-9, miR-134 and miR-191 were found to be dysregulated in HNSCC patient saliva compared to healthy controls; serving as a potential novel biomarker panel to detect HNSCC in a non-invasive manner [70].

In HPV-related HNSCC specifically, miR-34a is significantly down-regulated as the viral-protein E6 destabilizes p53 [70]. It was revealed later that the cross-talk between miR-34a and p53 plays a major role as tumour suppressor [70]. As transcriptional target of p53, miR-34a induces cell cycle arrest and apoptosis [70]. miR-34a therefore, could be incorporated into potential miRNA HNSCC biomarker panel to determine the HPV status of of a person [70]. Other lesser known dysregulated miRNA in HPV-related HNSCC include miR-125a, miR-126, miR-127-3p, miR142-5p, miR-145, miR-155, miR-181a, miR-181a, miR-181b, miR-20b, miR-218, miR-221, miR-222, miR-24a, miR-29a, miR-33, miR-363, miR-379, miR-497, miR-15a, miR-145, miR-20b, miR-21, miR-127-3p and miR-224 [70].

7. Current and Future Trends in the Treatment of Head and Neck Cancers

Open surgery remains as the first-line of treatment for HNSCC patients followed by chemotherapy and radiation [92]. It is the primary treatment for HNSCC in the oral cavity and salivary glands [92]. Open surgery is a popular choice for HNSCC patients living in developing countries because of the poor socioeconomic status and cannot afford advanced treatments [92]. There are two types of open surgeries currently in clinical practice depending on the severity of the tumour [93]. Tumours with tumour circumference smaller than 2cm would usually receive a negative surgical margin (complete removal of the cancer cells) while tumour with circumference larger than 2cm would usually receive a positive surgical margin (fragmentary removal of the cancer cells) to prevent the impairment of vital functions such as speech, chewing and ingesting [93]. The risk of open surgery has decreased significantly for the past decade as technology progress [92]. Inventions such as image-guided surgery and robotics increase the accuracy and precision of the operation, minimizing deformity to allow a better quality of life [92].

(i) Oral Cavity

Generally the treatment for oral cavity cancer is surgery to the primary lesion and to the necks. High dose radiotherapy to the mouth is regarded as very morbid with significant complications of a dry mouth and dental sepsis which can lead on to osteoradionecrosis [94]. Transoral resections, the splitting of the lip for access, or dropping the tongue into the neck are ways of accessing mouth cancers. Frequently part of the jaw needs to be removed. In general, radiotherapy is given post-operatively if a tongue primary has more than 7-10 mm depth invasion. A 5mm cancer depth generally indicates a 15% chance of microscopic nodal disease, while a 10mm depth or higher indicates a 30% chance of subclinical nodal disease [95]. Generally the nodes are best treated if there is a 15% or more chance of later neck disease, bearing in mind the complications of such treatment are not insignificant. Chemotherapy is added to radiotherapy if the primary has positive margins on surgical excision, or the lymph nodes show histological evidence of extracapsular spread.

There is emerging evidence that chronic irritation is a causative factor in oral cavity cancer. It seems to be especially important in young women [96]. Twenty percent of mouth cancers occur in lifelong non-smokers, generally in areas of chronic dental trauma [97]. Flap reconstruction has improved with the buccinator flap being used for small lateral defects. Radial forearm and anterior thigh flaps are used for bigger reconstructions. The fibula and hip bone are used for large reconstructions of the jaw and when there may be a role for later dental implants, especially if the reconstructed bone hasn't needed radiotherapy [98].

(ii) Oropharynx

Oropharyngeal cancers have seen the most changes in the last twenty years. There is an emerging trend in developing countries for the HPV to be involved in the carcinogenesis of oropharyngeal SCC, especially in smokers and ex-smokers. At our clinic in the last ten years nearly four hundred people have presented with oral cavity cancer and four hundred with oropharyngeal cancer. Lifelong non-smokers comprised 22% of the oral cavity group and 14% of the oropharyngeal group [97]. Of these, very few non-smoking women had oropharyngeal tumours, but women made up the majority of the oral cancer non-smokers. The incidence of HPV associated cancers is rising and in lifelong non-smokers HPV associated oropharyngeal cancer may well overtake oral cavity cancer. Around 80-90% of oropharyngeal malignancies now have HPV as a factor in their carcinogenesis and in their treatment paradigm. It is hoped that the Gardasil vaccine given to boys will stop this emerging cancer in decades to come. At present however, the incidence of HPV oropharyngeal cancer is now rising at about 2% per year [99].

Chemoradiotherapy has seen cure rates of above 90% for HPV associated oropharyngeal cancers in the lifelong non-smokers, even for the larger tumours [100].The cure rate for the HPV negative tumours – nearly always in smokers – is still quite low, possibly even as low as half those cure rate figures [101]. The cure rate of HPV associated oropharyngeal tumours is so high that there is a move to de-escalate therapy. Tonsil cancers when small and lateralised can often be dealt with by simply treating the lymph nodes on the ipsilateral side. Some centres are also doing this for small, well-lateralised base of tongue tumours [102]. When the nodes are bigger than 4cm, there is a tendency to treat lymph nodes in both sides of the neck. An emerging trend is to use the PET CT scan as an indicator of successful therapy and the PET CT is done four months after treatment is finished [103]. If there is a significant improvement in the amount of PET avidity in the primary site and neck nodes, that PET CT is repeated four to six weeks later. If there's minimal activity there is ongoing observation of the neck nodes with CT scans, but if there is residual activity a salvage neck dissection is performed often with the need for a pectoralis major flap or similar flap to reinforce the skin after the neck dissection to stop wound breakdown, exposure of the carotid artery and carotid artery blowout. When patients don't survive this cancer it's either due to distant metastatic spread to the liver, lungs and sometimes bones, or uncontrollable neck node disease after chemoradiotherapy. Normally the primary tumour is readily controlled with chemoradiotherapy, but nodes and metastases are harder to cure.

There's an emerging role for transoral resection of the small oropharyngeal tumours using either laser or robotic surgical techniques [104-106]. If clear margins can be obtained and the neck node burden is light, the patients may simply be treated with single modality surgical treatment. There's an emerging trend for the bigger primaries and bigger nodal burdens to have de-escalated therapy, having 50 - 55 Gray of radiotherapy rather than 65 - 72 Gray in the unoperated neck. However this de-escalation of therapy is very controversial and needs to be done in a controlled way. Overshooting de-escalation will decrease survival.

(iii) Nasopharynx

Nasopharyngeal carcinoma is very common in East Asian people and is associated with the Epstein Barr virus. The mainstay of treatment is chemoradiotherapy. For very large tumours induction chemotherapy is sometimes given. There is a limited role for surgery for small nasopharyngeal tumours that may recur [107, 108]. It's unusual for it to be used as the primary treatment modality. Some nasal and nasopharyngeal tumours are associated with HPV and would expect to do reasonably well with radiotherapy, but the Ebstein Barr virus tumours seem to respond quite well considering they often present with penetration of skull base and lymph node involvement at multiple levels. There are vaccine trials and novel drugs being trialled in various centres [109].

(iv) Larynx

Laryngeal treatment is very much associated with the organ-sparing techniques of radiotherapy or chemoradiotherapy. The initial VA study showed very high cure rates with high dose chemoradiotherapy over previous treatment protocols using the lower doses and that has resulted in many fewer laryngectomies and partial laryngectomies [110, 111]. However it has been shown that laryngeal cancer cure rates have, if anything, fallen over time [112]. The original VA study showed high incidence of trachesotomies and percutaneous gastrostomy feeding tubes being required post this non-surgical treatment and this has led to some controversy as to when this treatment should be given. There is a move for lasers to be used on small glottic cancers to avoid radiotherapy. Chemoradiotherapy is the standard treatment for intermediate size tumours, but there are transoral resection modalities using laser or robotic machines for the smaller and moderate sized supraglottic tumours. Laryngectomy is still used for the large tumours where there is an incompetent larynx or wide laryngeal cartilage involvement.

(v) Hypopharynx

Hypopharynx is regarded as generally as a surgical disease although there have been good results with chemoradiotherapy from Toronto. Our own clinic uses pharyngolaryngectomy with jejunal replacement as the standard therapy, and compares other treatments to that. For smaller tumours or at patient request chemoradiotherapy is given and we are yet to see what those figures are like. With surgery in our hands five year survival rate is in the order of 65% [113]. Other departments use tube skin flaps or stomach pull-ups. Hypopharynx is regarded as an aggressive cancer and not particularly radiosensitive [114].The transoral robotic surgery may well find a place here for the very small tumours.

(vi) Neck Disease

The highly selective neck dissections are getting to be more the norm. Instead of the full radical neck dissection taking the sternomastoid muscle, internal jugular vein and accessory nerve, the standard operation for most head and neck cancer procedures is a II-IV neck dissection, sometimes taking level 1 for something anterior in the upper airway and level V possibly for something more posterior. If there's a midline primary tumour both necks need to be addressed. Generally we look at treatment to the other side of the neck if a node is bigger than 4cm suggesting there could be retrograde spread, or there's been previous radiotherapy or surgery to the neck. There is an emerging trend to take the lingual tonsils off the base of tongue, sometimes called a tongue base mucosectomy, to identify primary tumour site of origin when traditional tonsillectomy and panendoscopy with biopsy have been unsuccessful. This is especially so when the nodal disease is p16 positive [115-117].

(vii) Excision Repair Cross-Complementation Group 1

Excision Repair Cross-Complementation Group 1 (ERCC1) protein plays a significant role in the repair of DNA damage caused by platinum agents and is useful in identifying patients who will benefit from platinum based therapy. The mode of action of platinum based therapies is by creating DNA adducts which inhibit DNA replication and transcription in cancer cells. Preliminary data demonstrates that ERCC1 has a role in predicting patient responders to cisplatin based therapy in HNSCC. In a study by Handra-Luca et al, where ERCC1 was measured by IHC in 96 pre-treatment tissue samples 71% had high ERCC1 expression. The study found that pre-treatment ERCC1 expression levels inversely correlated with response and survival following cisplating based therapy. In further studies, low ERCC1 patients were found to have longer 3 year progression free survival (PFS) than those with high expression of ERCC1 (83.3% vs 49.4%). The 3 year overall survival (OS) was also found to be significantly higher in patients with low ERCC1 expression (91.7% vs 45.5%).

The clinical relevance of ERCC1 is yet to be validated, however it shows significant progress. High ERCC1 expression in HNSCC tumours can suggest poor platinum-based therapy responses and a probably switch to non-platinum based therapies.

(viii) Ribonucleotide Reductase M1

The Ribonucleotide Reductase M1 (RRM1) gene codes for a regulatory subunit of the enzyme ribonucleotide reductase which is a molecular target of a nucleoside analogue used for chemotherapy, Gemcitabine.

Pre-clinical studies have demonstrated that elevated levels or mutations in RRM1 have been attributed to gemcitabine resistance. Further studies are warranted to determine the role of RRM1 in determining the chemosensitivity in HNSCC.

(ix) β-Tubulin

In HNSCC, docetaxel in combination with cisplatin and 5-fluorouracil (5-FU) has become part of the standard induction regimen. Taxanes mode of action in anticancer activity works by binding to β-tubulin polymers and inhibiting microtubule depolymerisation as well as mitotic progression. In a phase 3 trial comparing induction with 5-FU to induction with cisplatin and 5-FU showed that β-tubulin II as measured by IHC is associated with clinical outcomes. In 265 patients out of 501, patients with low β-tubulin II expression had better PFS and OS. In this subset of the patient cohort, there was greater benefit from the addition of docetaxel to the induction therapy. In the high β-tubulin II expression groups, there were negligible differences as per the 2 induction regimens. The use of taxanes in HNSCC is increasing and therefore, the clinical utility of β-tubulin isoforms may play an important role for therapeutic purposes.

(x) Palliation

Palliation is an important part of HNC treatment. Hypofractionated regimens of four, six or twenty treatments over four weeks are sometimes used in patients to just get local control for a year or two with minimal side effects from that radiotherapy while the disease takes its course; either in the head and neck cancer disease with metastasis or the patient being very elderly or infirm from other conditions. Palliative chemotherapy may have a part to play and Gemcitabine, Cisplatinum and Taxol medications seem to have a role in this.

8. Companies That Are Active in Salivary Diagnostics and Head and Neck Cancers

I. Oasis Diagnostics ® Corporation

Oasis Diagnostics ® Corporation is a company founded in 2002 which has pioneered saliva based technologies for rapid screening, sample collection and molecular diagnostics. The company understands that early detection and non-invasive diagnostics are key for disease prevention globally and aims to push the boundaries to improve the quality of healthcare [118]. The company has a specialized proprietary range of products ranging from oral fluid rapid test platforms, oral fluid collection devices, salivary DNA collection devices, universal saliva collection devices as well as novel products for RNA/protein collection for genomic/proteomic studies [119].

II. Forsyth

Forsyth is an institute founded in 2013, which has attracted over 4 million dollars in funding for salivary diagnostics. The broad scope of this institute is to provide a simple non-invasive test which could one day replace blood based methods. The institute envisages a medical diagnostics world where salivary tests could provide valuable information pertaining to systemic diseases. The institute has currently four keen areas that involve salivary diagnostic applications and include salivary biomarkers that can predict pre-diabetes/metabolic syndrome. An active tuberculosis (TB) project which aims to distinguish active TB from the latent or inactive state and is supported by the Bill & Melinda Gates Foundation. Progressive periodontitis project which aims to identify individuals who have progressive disease allowing clinicians to better treat the patients and finally, the Inflammatory profile project which aims to identify salivary biomarkers that can identify individuals at a higher risk of heart disease, stroke, Type 2 diabetes and Alzheimer's disease to name a few [120].

III. ViennaLab Diagnostics

ViennaLab Diagnostics based in Austria and produces simple in vitro diagnostic kits for the detection of genetic mutations, methylation status and genetic predispositions. Amongst their products are genetic tests which can identify oncogene mutations which can inform the best approach for treatment, such as somatic mutations in the epidermal growth factor receptor tyrosine kinase (EGFR-TK) which can influence the treatment by EGFR-TK inhibitors. The assays identify the most prevalent mutations relevant for anti EGFR-TK therapy. Other oncology assays that the company focus are mutations assays for KRAS & NRAS, PGC-5FU, PGXX-TMPT, BRAF and FCGR [121].

IV. Proteocyte Diagnostics

Proteocycte Diagnostics Inc is a company from Canada which develops novel diagnostic technologies for management of HNCs.Their products include Straticyte™ assay to determine the risk of oral premalignant lesions transforming into cancers. This company identified proteins by comparing HNCs tumour tissue with normal tissue. The Straticyte™ test uses antibodies to determine and quantity cancer biomarkers and also by referencing to databases allows them to score the progression risk of a lesion. This technology took over 10 years of research, has over 7 peer reviewed publications and is protected by 5 patent applications [122].

V. Navidea Biopharmaceuticals

Navida Biopharmaceuticals is a leading diagnostics company that aims to pinpoint molecular sites and pathways to identify disease states. A recent product by the company, Lymphoseek® (technetium Tc 99m tilmanocept) is the first FDA approved sentinel lymph node biopsy agent for use in HNC patients and oral cavity carcinoma. Conventional standard care for HNC patients include the removal of multiple lymph nodes during a surgical procedure. Whereas, sentinel lymph node mapping could provide an effective alternative to elective neck dissection. As a result of this, Lymphoseek® has the potential to more easily stage cancers and direct surgical treatment thereby improving patient survival [123].

VI. Zenalux Biomedical

Zenalux Biomedical, a leader in biophotonic diagnostics has in collaborations with Roswell Park Cancer Institute (RPCI) developed the Zenascope PC1 system which allows basic quantitative spectroscopy, pressure sensing, imaging and illumination. With their collaborative efforts, the company aims to design a system able to detect oral cancers at an early stage. The new preclinical, Zenascope IM1 system aims to compliment imaging with spectrographic data as well as provide better visualization of cellular changes and tumour margins. The instrument works by shining a white light onto opaque target media and measure and analyses the reflected signals. The system is able to provide targeted endpoints to haemoglobin concentration, saturation and scattering as a measure of cell density and necrosis to name a few. Other areas of interest where the device is currently being used is in accelerated feedback in drug discovery, response to therapy, breast tumour margin assessment, breast biopsy and cervical cancer detection [124].

9. The Future Perspectives

Whilst HNSCC stands as the six most common cancer worldwide, the incidence rate is on the decline in the western world [125]. Since majority of the big pharma companies are situated in the western world, they are less interested in developing new drugs for HNSCC [125]. As a result, there is no new therapy in the pipeline; causing HNSCC to fall into the category of 'neglected disease' [125]. In addition, the development of the new targeted therapies for HNSCC requires larger investments and is also time consuming, an effective way to solve this unmet clinical need is to merge existing HNSCC disease causing targets with existing drugs [125]. This strategy bypasses the discovery and validation phase that are required by pharma companies when introducing new drug targets into clinical trials to discern to efficacy and safety [125]. As 50% of all new drugs fail under the safety aspect, said method not only decreases the expenses and development time but also the risk of getting rejected due to safety issue [125].

Early diagnosis and good prognosis decreases the mortality rate due to HNSCC [90, 126, 127]. As such, biomarkers with the power to diagnose and prognosis the disease are invaluable. Many HNSCC biomarkers have been discovered, however, these data need to be integrated into patient care for these to be valuable [128]. Conversely, the focus should not fall solely on diagnostic and prognostic biomarkers; predictive biomarkers are just as important to determine the ideal treatment response in HNSCC patients [128]. For example in HPV-negative HNSCC patients, the focus revolved around the improvement of patient survival [128]. With regards to this subject matter, the presence of predictive biomarkers would be beneficial in patient selection for precise therapeutic treatment; assisting in better therapeutic window estimation [128].

The future for molecular screening requires a close collaboration between imaging and biomarker-based investigations. While biomarkers will have the ability to provide quantifiable characteristics, imaging will provide temporal and special features of the disease space and amplify biomarker visualization in real time. Smart reagents and probes are needed to exploit the power of imaging, and biomarkers could provide some needed probes. A comprehensive database of biomarkers needs to be developed, integrating genomics, proteomics, metabolomics, glycomics, and imaging features of a broad spectrum of disease states. As technologies continue to mature, reference reagents and samples must be made available to investigators to provide standards for their exploratory studies and allow for consistencies in cross-validation among studies. However, standards should not be imposed in the initial discovery phase that could impede innovations. The future could well be involved with small molecules, circulating tumour cells and novel markers suggesting different treatments are required [36, 129]. Tropical plant agents and Taxols come into play. Intensity Modulated Radiotherapy and Proton Therapy are emerging. The free availability of reconstruction options in our department has led on to a pectoralis major flap frequently being used to reinforce suture lines in necks which have been irradiated. Free flap reconstructions are the standard, although sometimes we get away with a buccinator flap or local flap. Earlier diagnosis would be ideal as smaller tumours have a better prognosis. Blood and saliva tests for markers of respiratory and HNCs may emerge [70].

In order to move forward the fields of early diagnosis, prognosis and risk stratification in HNSCC patients, communications and integration between basic researchers and clinicians is highly warranted [128]. Both professions need to work closely together to better interpret the laboratory data and translate them into useful clinical information [128]. Therefore, it is highly recommended that clinicians should educate themselves to understand the basic principle of the technology used in the laboratory and their respective limitations [128]. We forecast that in the next few years, there will be early diagnostic strategies in place for HNSCC whereby improving patient care and management whereby significantly reducing the mortalities and morbidities associated with this devastating disease.

Acknowledgments

This work is supported by the Garnett Passe & Rodney Williams Memorial Foundation, QUT start-up grant and the Queensland Centre for Head and Neck Cancer funded by Atlantic Philanthropies, the Queensland Government and the Princess Alexandra Hospital. We also thank Mr. Roberto Chata for helping us with figure illustrations.

References

[1] van Monsjou, H.S., et al., Head and neck squamous cell carcinoma in young patients. *Oral Oncol,* 2013. 49(12): p. 1097-102.

[2] Argiris, A., et al., Head and neck cancer. *Lancet,* 2008. 371(9625): p. 1695-709.

[3] Wyss, A., et al., Cigarette, cigar, and pipe smoking and the risk of head and neck cancers: pooled analysis in the International Head and Neck Cancer Epidemiology Consortium. *Am J Epidemio*l, 2013. 178(5): p. 679-90.

[4] Markopoulou, S., G. Nikolaidis, and T. Liloglou, DNA methylation biomarkers in biological fluids for early detection of respiratory tract cancer. *Clin Chem Lab Med,* 2012. 50(10): p. 1723-31.

[5] Arantes, L.M., et al., Methylation as a biomarker for head and neck cancer. *Oral Oncol,* 2014. 50(6): p. 587-92.

[6] Galbiatti, A.L., et al., Head and neck cancer: causes, prevention and treatment. *Braz J Otorhinolaryngol*, 2013. 79(2): p. 239-47.

[7] Weiss, D., et al., Protein expression and promoter methylation of the candidate biomarker TCF21 in head and neck squamous cell carcinoma. *Cell Oncol* (Dordr), 2013. 36(3): p. 213-24.

[8] Lam, L., et al., Retrospective study of survival and treatment pattern in a cohort of patients with oral and oropharyngeal tongue cancers from 1987 to 2004. *Oral Oncol,* 2007. 43(2): p. 150-8.

[9] Mashberg, A. and A. Samit, Early diagnosis of asymptomatic oral and oropharyngeal squamous cancers. *CA Cancer J Clin,* 1995. 45(6): p. 328-51.

[10] Mydlarz, W.K., P.T. Hennessey, and J.A. Califano, Advances and Perspectives in the Molecular Diagnosis of Head and Neck Cancer. *Expert opinion on medical diagnostics,* 2010. 4(1): p. 53-65.

[11] Tran, N., et al., Potential role of micro-RNAs in head and neck tumorigenesis. *Head Neck,* 2010. 32(8): p. 1099-111.

[12] Barnes, L., et al., Pathology and genetics of head and neck tumours. *IARC Press,* Lyon, 2005.

[13] D'Souza, G. and A. Dempsey, The role of HPV in head and neck cancer and review of the HPV vaccine. *Prev Med,* 2011. 53 Suppl 1: p. S5-S11.

[14] Brakenhoff, R.H., Cancer. Another NOTCH for cancer. *Science,* 2011. 333(6046): p. 1102-3.

[15] Han, S., et al., Epidemiology and cost analysis for patients with oral cancer in a university hospital in China. *BMC Public Health*, 2010. 10: p. 196.

[16] Lee, K.D., H.S. Lee, and C.H. Jeon, Body fluid biomarkers for early detection of head and neck squamous cell carcinomas. *Anticancer Res,* 2011. 31(4): p. 1161-7.

[17] Ndiaye, C., et al., HPV DNA, E6/E7 mRNA, and p16INK4a detection in head and neck cancers: a systematic review and meta-analysis. *The Lancet Oncology,* 2014. 15(12): p. 1319-1331.

[18] Oliveira, M.C., et al., Epidemiology of HPV in head and neck cancer. *InTech,* 2012.

[19] Australian Institute of Health and Welfare 2014, Head and neck cancers in Australia. Cancer Series no. 83, 2014.

[20] Humber and Yorkshire Coast Cancer Network, HYCCN guidelines for management of adult patients with head and neck cancers version 1.2. Humber and Yorkshire Coast Cancer Network, 2011.

[21] Dwojak, S.M. and N. Bhattacharyya, Incremental and comparative health care expenditures for head and neck cancer in the United States. *Laryngoscope,* 2014. 124(10): p. 2305-8.

[22] Pulte, D. and H. Brenner, Changes in survival in head and neck cancers in the late 20th and early 21st century: a period analysis. *Oncologist,* 2010. 15(9): p. 994-1001.

[23] Kulkarni, M.R., Head and neck cancer burden in India. *IJHNS,* 2013. 4(1): p. 29-35.

[24] Bhattacharjee, A., A. Chakraborty, and P. Purkaystha, Prevalence of head and neck cancers in the north east—An institutional study. *Indian Journal of Otolaryngology and Head & Neck Surgery,* 2006. 58(1): p. 15-19.

[25] Agrawal, N., et al., Exome Sequencing of Head and Neck Squamous Cell Carcinoma Reveals Inactivating Mutations in NOTCH1. *Science,* 2011. 333(6046): p. 1154-1157.

[26] Stransky, N., et al., The Mutational Landscape of Head and Neck Squamous Cell Carcinoma. *Science,* 2011. 333(6046): p. 1157-1160.

[27] Riaz, N., et al., Unraveling the molecular genetics of head and neck cancer through genome-wide approaches. *Genes & Diseases,* 2014. 1(1): p. 75-86.

[28] Vogelstein, B., D. Lane, and A.J. Levine, Surfing the p53 network. *Nature*, 2000. 408(6810): p. 307-310.

[29] Bolt, J., et al., The ATM/p53 pathway is commonly targeted for inactivation in squamous cell carcinoma of the head and neck (SCCHN) by multiple molecular mechanisms. *Oral Oncol,* 2005. 41(10): p. 1013-20.

[30] Rubin Grandis, J., Q. Zeng, and D.J. Tweardy, Retinoic acid normalizes the increased gene transcription rate of TGF-alpha and EGFR in head and neck cancer cell lines. *Nat Med,* 1996. 2(2): p. 237-40.

[31] Kalyankrishna, S. and J.R. Grandis, Epidermal growth factor receptor biology in head and neck cancer. *J Clin Oncol,* 2006. 24(17): p. 2666-72.

[32] Sok, J.C., et al., Mutant epidermal growth factor receptor (EGFRvIII) contributes to head and neck cancer growth and resistance to EGFR targeting. *Clin Cancer Res,* 2006. 12(17): p. 5064-73.

[33] Klein, J.D. and J.R. Grandis, The molecular pathogenesis of head and neck cancer. *Cancer biology & therapy,* 2010. 9(1): p. 1-7.

[34] Park, B.J., S.I. Chiosea, and J.R. Grandis, Molecular changes in the multistage pathogenesis of head and neck cancer. *Cancer biomarkers : section A of Disease markers,* 2010. 9(1-6): p. 325-339.

[35] Hoa, M., et al., Amplification of wild-type K-ras promotes growth of head and neck squamous cell carcinoma. *Cancer research,* 2002. 62(24): p. 7154-7156.

[36] Kulasinghe, A., et al., Circulating Tumour Cells in Metastatic Head and Neck Cancers. *Int J Cancer,* 2014.

[37] Palka, K.T., R.J. Slebos, and C.H. Chung, Update on Molecular Diagnostic Tests in Head and Neck Cancer. *Seminars in oncology,* 2008. 35(3): p. 198-210.

[38] Warnakulasuriya, S., Global epidemiology of oral and oropharyngeal cancer. *Oral Oncol,* 2009. 45(4-5): p. 309-16.

[39] Sujatha, D., P.B. Hebbar, and A. Pai, Prevalence and correlation of oral lesions among tobacco smokers, tobacco chewers, areca nut and alcohol users. *Asian Pac J Cancer Prev,* 2012. 13(4): p. 1633-7.

[40] Board, C.N.E. Head and Neck Cancer: Diagnosis. 2014; Available from: http://www.cancer.net/cancer-types/head-and-neck-cancer/diagnosis.

[41] D'Souza, G., et al., Case-control study of human papillomavirus and oropharyngeal cancer. *N Engl J Med,* 2007. 356(19): p. 1944-56.

[42] Zhang, H.S., A.A. Postigo, and D.C. Dean, Active transcriptional repression by the Rb-E2F complex mediates G1 arrest triggered by p16INK4a, TGFbeta, and contact inhibition. *Cell,* 1999. 97(1): p. 53-61.

[43] Mendelsohn, A.H., et al., Histopathologic findings of HPV and p16 positive HNSCC. *Laryngoscope,* 2010. 120(9): p. 1788-94.

[44] Robinson, M., P. Sloan, and R. Shaw, Refining the diagnosis of oropharyngeal squamous cell carcinoma using human papillomavirus testing. *Oral Oncol,* 2010. 46(7): p. 492-6.

[45] Lewis, J.S., Jr., et al., p16 positive oropharyngeal squamous cell carcinoma:an entity with a favorable prognosis regardless of tumor HPV status. *Am J Surg Pathol,* 2010. 34(8): p. 1088-96.

[46] Hoffmann, M., et al., HPV DNA, E6*I-mRNA expression and p16INK4A immunohistochemistry in head and neck cancer - how valid is p16INK4A as surrogate marker? *Cancer Lett,* 2012. 323(1): p. 88-96.

[47] Harris, S.L., et al., Association of p16(INK4a) overexpression with improved outcomes in young patients with squamous cell cancers of the oral tongue. *Head Neck,* 2011. 33(11): p. 1622-7.

[48] Liang, C., et al., Biomarkers of HPV in head and neck squamous cell carcinoma. *Cancer Res,* 2012. 72(19): p. 5004-13.

[49] Lewis, J.S., Jr., p16 Immunohistochemistry as a standalone test for risk stratification in oropharyngeal squamous cell carcinoma. *Head Neck Pathol,* 2012. 6 Suppl 1: p. S75-82.

[50] Ferlito, A., et al., Changing concepts in the surgical management of the cervical node metastasis. 2003, *Elsevier Ltd:* England. p. 429-435.

[51] Takes, R.P., Staging of the neck in patients with head and neck squamous cell cancer: Imaging techniques and biomarkers. *Oral oncology,* 2004. 40(7): p. 656-667.

[52] van Wilgen, C.P., et al., Shoulder complaints after nerve sparing neck dissections. *Int J Oral Maxillofac Surg,* 2004. 33(3): p. 253-7.

[53] Roigo, J.P., et al., Can biomarkers play a role in the decision about treatment of the clinically negative neck in patients with head and neck cancer? *Head and Neck-Journal for the Sciences and Specialties of the Head and Neck,* 2008. 30(4): p. 525-538.

[54] Nichols, A.C., et al., Detection of circulating tumor cells in advanced head and neck cancer using the CellSearch system. *Head & neck,* 2012. 34(10): p. 1440-1444.

[55] Trials, C. Circulating Tumor Cells as an Early Predictive head-and -Neck Squamous-cell Carcinoma (CIRCUTEC). 2014 [cited 2014; Available from: http://clinicaltrials.gov/show/NCT02119559.

[56] Institute, N.C. Stage Information for Breast Cancer 2014 [cited 2014 01/12/2014]; Available from: http://www.cancer.gov/cancertopics/pdq /treatment/breast/health professional/page3.

[57] Speicher, M.R. and K. Pantel, Tumor signatures in the blood. *Nature biotechnology,* 2014. 32(5): p. 441-443.

[58] Bettegowda, C., et al., Detection of circulating tumor DNA in early and late stage human malignancies. *Neuro-oncology,* 2014. 16 Suppl 3(suppl 3): p. iii7-iii7.

[59] Zuo, J.-H., et al., Activation of EGFR promotes squamous carcinoma SCC10A cell migration and invasion via inducing EMT-like phenotype change and MMP-9-mediated degradation of E-cadherin. *Journal of cellular biochemistry,* 2011. 112(9): p. 2508-2517.

[60] Pantel, K. and C. Alix-Panabières, Real-time liquid biopsy in cancer patients: fact or fiction? *Cancer research,* 2013. 73(21): p. 6384-6388.

[61] INCHEM, I., Biomarkers in Risk Assessment: Validity and Validation. 2014.

[62] Institute, N.C., Biomarkers: the key to early detection. 2014.

[63] Wagner, P.D., M. Verma, and S. Srivastava, Challenges for biomarkers in cancer detection. Annals of the New York Academy of Sciences, 2004. 1022(1): p. 9-16.

[64] Zhang, Y., et al., The emerging landscape of salivary diagnostics. *Oral Health Dent Manag,* 2014. 13(2): p. 200-10.

[65] Pepe, M.S., et al., Pivotal Evaluation of the Accuracy of a Biomarker Used for Classification or Prediction: Standards for Study Design. *Journal of the National Cancer Institute,* 2008. 100(20): p. 1432-1438.
[66] Ovchinnikov, D.A., et al., DNA Methylation at the Novel CpG Sites in the Promoter of MED15/PCQAP Gene as a Biomarker for Head and Neck Cancers. *Biomark Insights,* 2014. 9: p. 53-60.
[67] Pandit, P., J. Cooper-White, and C. Punyadeera, High-yield RNA-extraction method for saliva. *Clin Chem,* 2013. 59(7): p. 1118-22.
[68] Salazar, C., et al., A novel saliva-based microRNA biomarker panel to detect head and neck cancers. Cell Oncol (Dordr), 2014. 37(5): p. 331-8.
[69] Nagadia, R., et al., miRNAs in head and neck cancer revisited. *Cell Oncol* (Dordr), 2013. 36(1): p. 1-7.
[70] Salazar, C., D. Calvopina, and C. Punyadeera, miRNAs in human papilloma virus associated oral and oropharyngeal squamous cell carcinomas. *Expert Rev Mol Diagn,* 2014. 14(8): p. 1033-40.
[71] Ovchinnikov, D.A., et al., Tumor-suppressor Gene Promoter Hypermethylation in Saliva of Head and Neck Cancer Patients. *Translational Oncology,* 2012. 5(5): p. 321-6.
[72] Pfaffe, T., et al., Diagnostic potential of saliva: current state and future applications. *Clinical Chemistry,* 2011. 57(5): p. 675-87.
[73] Arabi, H., et al., Impact of microsatellite instability (MSI) on survival in high grade endometrial carcinoma. *Gynecol Oncol,* 2009. 113(2): p. 153-8.
[74] Stepanov, V.A., et al., [Analysis of genetic diversity of population of Northern Eurasia from autosomal microsatellite loci]. *Genetika*, 2003. 39(10): p. 1381-8.
[75] Stur, E., et al., Microsatellite Instability in Head and Neck Squamous Cell Carcinoma: A Study of a Brazilian Population. *ISRN Biomarkers,* 2013. 2013: p. 5.
[76] Chakrabarti, S., et al., Microsatellite instability in squamous cell carcinoma of head and neck from the Indian patient population. *Int J Cancer,* 2001. 92(4): p. 555-61.
[77] Sasiadek, M.M., et al., Impairment of MLH1 and CDKN2A in oncogenesis of laryngeal cancer. *Br J Cancer,* 2004. 90(8): p. 1594-9.
[78] Esteller, M., Epigenetics in cancer. *N Engl J Med,* 2008. 358(11): p. 1148-59.
[79] Singal, R. and G.D. Ginder, DNA methylation. *Blood*, 1999. 93(12): p. 4059-70.
[80] Momparler, R.L. and V. Bovenzi, DNA methylation and cancer. *J Cell Physiol,* 2000. 183(2): p. 145-54.
[81] Carvalho, A.L., et al., Detection of promoter hypermethylation in salivary rinses as a biomarker for head and neck squamous cell carcinoma surveillance. *Clin Cancer Res,* 2011. 17(14): p. 4782-9.
[82] Kaur, J., et al., Promoter hypermethylation in Indian primary oral squamous cell carcinoma. International journal of cancer. *Journal international du cancer,* 2010. 127(10): p. 2367-2373.
[83] Nagata, S., et al., Aberrant DNA methylation of tumor-related genes in oral rinse: a noninvasive method for detection of oral squamous cell carcinoma. *Cancer,* 2012. 118(17): p. 4298-308.
[84] Pattani, K.M., et al., Endothelin receptor type B gene promoter hypermethylation in salivary rinses is independently associated with risk of oral cavity cancer and premalignancy. *Cancer Prev Res* (Phila), 2010. 3(9): p. 1093-103.

[85] Guerrero-Preston, R., et al., NID2 and HOXA9 promoter hypermethylation as biomarkers for prevention and early detection in oral cavity squamous cell carcinoma tissues and saliva. *Cancer Prev Res* (Phila), 2011. 4(7): p. 1061-72.

[86] Huang, P., et al., Behaviour of 5-hydroxymethylcytosine in bisulfite sequencing. *PLoS ONE,* 2010. 5(1).

[87] Licchesi, J.D.F., Methylation-spcific PCR. *DNA Methylation: Methods and Protocols 2nd edition,* 2009. 507: p. 305-323.

[88] Huang, Z., C.F. Bassil, and S.K. Murphy, Methylation-specific PCR. *Methods Mol Biol,* 2013. 1049: p. 75-82.

[89] Ovchinnikov, D.A., et al., DNA Methylation at the Novel CpG Sites in the Promoter of MED15/PCQAP Gene as a Biomarker for Head and Neck Cancers. *Biomarker Insights*, 2014. 9: p. 53-60.

[90] Ovchinnikov, D.A., et al., Tumor-suppressor Gene Promoter Hypermethylation in Saliva of Head and Neck Cancer Patients. *Translational Oncology,* 2012. 5(5): p. 321-326.

[91] Huang, Y.K., et al., DNA methylation of PAX1 as a biomarker for oral squamous cell carcinoma. *Clin Oral Investig,* 2014. 18(3): p. 801-8.

[92] Hartl, D.M., et al., Is open surgery for head and neck cancers truly declining? *Eur Arch Otorhinolaryngol,* 2013. 270(11): p. 2793-802.

[93] Haque, R., et al., Surgical margins and survival after head and neck cancer surgery. *BMC Ear Nose Throat Disord,* 2006. 6: p. 2.

[94] Gore, S.M., et al., Concurrent chemoradiotherapy compared with surgery and adjuvant radiotherapy for oral cavity squamous cell carcinoma. *Head Neck,* 2014.

[95] Ganly, I., S. Patel, and J. Shah, Early stage squamous cell cancer of the oral tongue--clinicopathologic features affecting outcome. *Cancer*, 2012. 118(1): p. 101-11.

[96] Dahlstrom, K.R., et al., Squamous cell carcinoma of the head and neck in never smoker-never drinkers: a descriptive epidemiologic study. *Head Neck,* 2008. 30(1): p. 75-84.

[97] Perry, B.J., et al., Sites of Origin of Oral Cavity Cancer in Nonsmokers vs Smokers: Possible Evidence of Dental Trauma Carcinogenesis and Its Importance Compared With Human Papillomavirus. *JAMA Otolaryngol Head Neck Surg,* 2014.

[98] Sclaroff, A., et al., Immediate mandibular reconstruction and placement of dental implants At the time of ablative surgery. *Oral Surgery, Oral Medicine, Oral Pathology,* 1994. 78(6): p. 711-717.

[99] Ariyawardana, A. and N.W. Johnson, Trends of lip, oral cavity and oropharyngeal cancers in Australia 1982-2008: overall good news but with rising rates in the oropharynx. *BMC cancer,* 2013. 13(1): p. 333-333.

[100] Hong, A.M., et al., Human papillomavirus modifies the prognostic significance of T stage and possibly N stage in tonsillar cancer. *Ann Oncol,* 2013. 24(1): p. 215-9.

[101] Fakhry, C., et al., Improved survival of patients with human papillomavirus-positive head and neck squamous cell carcinoma in a prospective clinical trial. *J Natl Cancer Inst,* 2008. 100(4): p. 261-9.

[102] Sinha, P., et al., Histologic and systemic prognosticators for local control and survival in margin negative transoral laser microsurgery-treated oral cavity squamous cell carcinoma. *Head Neck*, 2013.

[103] Porceddu, S.V., et al., Results of a prospective study of positron emission tomography-directed management of residual nodal abnormalities in node-positive head and neck cancer after definitive radiotherapy with or without systemic therapy. *Head Neck,* 2011. 33(12): p. 1675-82.

[104] Adelstein, D.J., et al., Transoral resection of pharyngeal cancer: summary of a National Cancer Institute Head and Neck Cancer Steering Committee Clinical Trials Planning Meeting, November 6-7, 2011, Arlington, Virginia. *Head Neck,* 2012. 34(12): p. 1681-703.

[105] Weinstein, G.S., et al., Transoral robotic surgery: radical tonsillectomy. *Arch Otolaryngol Head Neck Surg*, 2007. 133(12): p. 1220-6.

[106] Haughey, B.H., et al., Transoral laser microsurgery as primary treatment for advanced-stage oropharyngeal cancer: a United States multicenter study. *Head Neck*, 2011. 33(12): p. 1683-94.

[107] Wei, W.I., et al., Surgical salvage of persistent or recurrent nasopharyngeal carcinoma with maxillary swing approach - Critical appraisal after 2 decades. *Head Neck,* 2011. 33(7): p. 969-75.

[108] Wei, W.I. and W.K. Ho, Transoral robotic resection of recurrent nasopharyngeal carcinoma. Laryngoscope, 2010. 120(10): p. 2011-4.

[109] Smith, C. and R. Khanna, A new approach for cellular immunotherapy of nasopharyngeal carcinoma. *Oncoimmunology,* 2012. 1(8): p. 1440-1442.

[110] Induction chemotherapy plus radiation compared with surgery plus radiation in patients with advanced laryngeal cancer. The Department of Veterans Affairs Laryngeal Cancer Study Group. *N Engl J Med,* 1991. 324(24): p. 1685-90.

[111] Forastiere, A.A., et al., Concurrent chemotherapy and radiotherapy for organ preservation in advanced laryngeal cancer. *N Engl J Med*, 2003. 349(22): p. 2091-8.

[112] Hoffman, H.T., et al., Laryngeal cancer in the United States: changes in demographics, patterns of care, and survival. *Laryngoscope*, 2006. 116(9 Pt 2 Suppl 111): p. 1-13.

[113] Bova, R., et al., Total pharyngolaryngectomy for squamous cell carcinoma of the hypopharynx: a review. *Laryngoscope*, 2005. 115(5): p. 864-9.

[114] Wahlberg, P.C., et al., Carcinoma of the hypopharynx: analysis of incidence and survival in Sweden over a 30-year period. *Head Neck,* 1998. 20(8): p. 714-9.

[115] Patel, S.A., et al., Robotic surgery for primary head and neck squamous cell carcinoma of unknown site. *JAMA Otolaryngol Head Neck Surg,* 2013. 139(11): p. 1203-11.

[116] Graboyes, E.M., et al., Management of human papillomavirus-related unknown primaries of the head and neck with a transoral surgical approach. *Head Neck*, 2014.

[117] Galloway, T.J., et al., HPV Association and the Increasing Incidence of Unknown Primary Head-and-Neck Squamous Cell Carcinoma. I*nternational Journal of Radiation Oncology Biology Physics*. 88(2): p. 494.

[118] Kwok, R., Dental science: Oral observatory. *Nature,* 2012. 486(7401): p. 147-148.

[119] Diagnostics, O., Oasis Diagnostics - Overview. 2014.

[120] Forsyth, Salivary Diagnostics. 2014.

[121] Viennalab, 2014.

[122] Diagnostics, P., Straticyte Technology. 2014.

[123] Biopharmaceuticals, N., 2014.

[124] Institute, R.P.C., Zenalux Collaborates with Roswell Park Cancer Institute to Enhance Zenascope for Oral Cancer Detection. 2014.

[125] Kulkarni, P. and U. Saxena, Head and neck cancers, the neglected malignancies: present and future treatment strategies. *Expert Opin Ther Targets*, 2014. 18(4): p. 351-4.

[126] Walden, M.J. and N. Aygun, Head and neck cancer. *Semin Roentgenol,* 2013. 48(1): p. 75-86.

[127] Ralhan, R., How will increasing our knowledge of the head and neck cancer cells' secretome benefit head and neck squamous cell carcinoma patients? *Expert Rev Proteomics,* 2012. 9(2): p. 115-8.

[128] Kang, H., A. Kiess, and C.H. Chung, Emerging biomarkers in head and neck cancer in the era of genomics. *Nat Rev Clin Oncol,* 2014.

[129] Chin, D., et al., Alpha B-crystallin, a new independent marker for poor prognosis in head and neck cancer. *Laryngoscope,* 2005. 115(7): p. 1239-42.

In: Head and Neck Cancer
Editor: Madison R. Hall

ISBN: 978-1-63482-113-1

Chapter 5

Human Papillomavirus in Head and Neck Cancer: Detection Methods and Clinical Significance

Keziah John[1], Maryam Jessri[1] and Camile S. Farah[1,2*]
[1]Oral Oncology Research Program, UQ Centre for Clinical Research, The University of Queensland, Herston, Queensland, Australia
[2]The Australian Centre for Oral Oncology Research & Education, Brisbane, Queensland, Australia

Abstract

Head and neck squamous cell carcinoma (HNSCC), the sixth most common cancer in the world, is associated with risk factors such as the use of tobacco, alcohol, areca nut, and more recently apparent, chronic infection of human papillomavirus (HPV). HPV-positive HNSCC is associated with improved clinical outcomes despite presentation at more advanced stages. This article reviews the contribution of HPV to HNSCC development and tumorigenesis, and the current literature on HPV detection methods. It also discusses the role of microRNAs and epigenetic changes involved in HPV-positive tumours, its response to radiation therapy, and a discussion on prognosis.

Keywords: head and neck cancer, human papillomavirus, detection methods, microRNA, epigenetics, radiation, immune response

* Corresponding author: Professor Camile S Farah, The Australian Centre for Oral Oncology Research & Education (ACORE), PO Box 88, Royal Brisbane & Women's Hospital, Herston QLD 4029 Australia, Tel: +61 7 3012 8760, Fax: +61 7 3012 7960, Email: camile@oralmedpath.com.au

Introduction

Head and neck cancer (HNC), including cancers of lip, oral cavity, nasal cavity, paranasal sinuses, pharynx, larynx, oropharynx, hypopharynx, salivary glands, and local lymph nodes, is the sixth most common cancer in the world. [1] Most of these cancers arise from epithelium and are collectively termed head and neck squamous cell carcinoma (HNSCC) and occur more commonly in consumers of tobacco and alcoholic products. [2] Excessive exposure to UV radiation is implicated in the incidence of lip SCC, while in certain populations (such as in India where HNSCC accounts for 40% of all malignancies) the use of the areca nut and betel quid products are causative of HNSCC. [2] Chronic infection with the human papillomavirus (HPV) has been implicated in oropharyngeal carcinoma (OPSCC), and more recently shown to involve the oral cavity proper. [2-5] Combinations of aetiological and risk factors are shown to have a synergistic effect – for example, the attributable risk of oral cancer due to consumption of both tobacco and alcohol products is estimated to be more than 80%. [4, 6]

HPV-positive HNSCC has a predilection for the oropharynx based on the microanatomy of this region. The increasing evidence implicates HPV in tissue transformation leading to SCC. There are numerous detection methods for HPV infection yielding varying prevalence rates. It is important that studies should be assessed based on sampling, HPV detection method utilised, ethnicity, geographic location, sample size of subjects examined, and grouping of subjects based on anatomical regions of the upper aerodigestive tract. [7, 8] While detection of HPV E6/E7 mRNA by qRT-PCR or RNA ISH are appropriate methodologies, next generation sequencing (NGS) is now emerging as a strong contender in diagnostic technology. Future methods of detecting HPV-involved cases could use miR and epigenetic profiles. It has been shown that HPV-positive tumours characteristically have a higher nodal metastasis and lower T-stage at time of presentation which indicates a low proliferation rate and enhanced metastatic potential. [9, 10] These have been shown to be more sensitive to chemoradiation, and improved locoregional control consistently translating into improved overall and disease-free survival. [11-14] Currently, based on National Comprehensive Cancer Network (NCCN) guidelines, changes in standard treatment protocols for OPSCC are not recommended for HPV-positive cases. [15]

The Human Papillomavirus

HPV is a small virus with circular double-stranded DNA (about 8 kbp) and a non-enveloped capsid, entirely dependent on its host replication cycle. [16] Of its 8 open reading frames, two "late" genes produce capsid proteins (L1, L2) and six "early" genes encode for the E1, E2, E4, E5, E6, and E7 proteins. [16] Over 200 genotypes of HPV have been identified. [16] Types -16, -18, -31, -33, and -45, amongst others, have been strongly implicated in malignant transformation of epithelial host cells and are termed high risk HPV (HR-HPV). [8, 16-18] Low risk HPV (genotypes -6, -11, -13 and -32) have been associated with benign oral proliferative epithelial lesions, squamous papilloma, common wart (verrucous vulgaris), condyloma acuminatum, and focal epithelial hyperplasia (Heck disease), which rarely become cancerous. [7, 19]

The reported prevalence of HPV in oral and oropharyngeal premalignant and malignant lesions ranges from 0% to 100%, owing to differences in sampling, HPV detection methods, ethnicity, geographic location, sample size of subjects examined, and inconsistent grouping of subjects with different lesions in different anatomical regions of the upper aerodigestive tract. [7, 8]

HPV Detection Methods

Determination of HPV status for OSCC and OPSCC will soon become the standard of care and is currently recommended by a number of organizations such as the National Comprehensive Cancer Network and The College of American Pathologists. [20, 21] The understanding of HPV oncogenesis is dependent on the local viral load and viral distribution, the clonality of HPV infection, the mechanism of HPV oncogene transcription, and the specific site of viral integration. [22] For decades, HPV could not be propagated in tissue culture, therefore in most cases the accurate identification of HPV relies on complex and multifaceted molecular biology techniques. [23, 24] The following is a brief description of current methodologies used to test for HPV DNA, RNA, and other surrogate markers of HPV.

A. Detection of Proteins

A.1. Immunohistochemistry (IHC)

Immunological detection of HPV proteins in human tissues has been hindered by the lack of sensitive and specific antibodies against viral proteins. [23] Furthermore while the early capsid proteins have a very low expression level, the late capsid proteins are only expressed in productive infections such as warts and they do not discriminate between HPV types. [23] Cyclin-dependent kinase inhibitor 2A (CDKN2A) encodes several transcript variants which differ in their first exon. A CDKN2A gene product, p16, is often used as a surrogate marker for HPV status as it is typically overexpressed in HPV-positive OSCC, however it is recommended that it not be relied on solely but be used in conjunction with HPV DNA or RNA detection. [21, 25] Bishop et al., [12] warn against p16 testing alone since a direct and mechanistic link between DNA integration and p16 expression cannot be established, and state that in sites that have not been confirmed as preferentially targeted by HPV (e.g. larynx, hypopharynx), it was unlikely that p16 overexpression reflects the presence of transcriptionally active HPV (i.e. low positive predictive value).

Lingen et al., [26] reported 79.2% sensitivity, 92.0% specificity, and a negative-predictive value of 98.6% for p16 IHC, but noted a poor positive-predictive value (41.3%) for HR-HPV E6/7 expression in OSCC. Bussu et al., [27] found immunoexpression of p16 to be a fair, but not excellent, diagnostic assay only in the oropharynx, which also displayed the highest HR-HPV infection rate, while Poling et al., [28] reported that p16 staining was not a reliable marker for transcriptionally active HPV in SCCs of the lateral tongue. Shi et al., [29] found 92% concordance between IHC and in situ hybridization (ISH), 86% concordance with HPV-16 E6 mRNA qRT-PCR and IHC, and 86% concordance between HPV16 ISH and E6 mRNA qRT-PCR, showing that qRT-PCR or ISH are both reasonable duplex methods. While there has been some debate over whether p16 expression specifically reflects HPV activity in OPSCC, [30] Gao et al., [31] concluded that p16 detection by IHC can be used as a highly sensitive and specific marker for HPV activity in OPSCC. The key advantage of IHC is that no specialized equipment or tissue handling is required, which is in stark contrast to Southern blot hybridization, ISH, PCR, and RT-PCR. [25]

A.2. Western Blot

Western blot uses gel electrophoresis to separate denatured proteins based on the length of their polypeptide or the 3-dimensional structure of native proteins. [23] Proteins are transferred to a nitrocellulose or polyvinylidene fluoride membrane and subsequently the protein of interest is identified by immunostaining. [23] Antibodies against early capsid proteins of HPV have been used to indirectly visualize these proteins in cell extracts but their use is mostly restricted to in-vitro assays. [23] Wang et al., [32] used Western blot and RT-PCR to detect HPV16/18 E6 and HPV18 E7 in human cell lines and discovered Western blot to be consistent with RT-PCR results. Compared to IHC, Western blot provides a more general overview of the cell population and accordingly requires a higher amount of protein input. [33] Western blot is time consuming and labour intensive; however, it has been shown to be highly consistent with ELISA in identifying different isotopes of early capsids of HPV16. [33]

B. Detection of HPV Nucleic Acids

B.1. Southern Blot

The Southern blot may be used to measure the number of copies of a given gene or to analyze DNA that is too repetitive for PCR amplification or other sequencing methods. [25] The procedure is labour intensive requiring the isolation of large amounts of highly purified genomic DNA, digestion with restriction endonucleases, separation of DNA by electrophoresis, transfer of DNA to nitrocellulose membrane, synthesis of radio-labelled nucleic acid probe(s), hybridization, and exposure of the film. [25] In addition, hybridization in solid phase, such as Southern blot for DNA and Northern blot for viral RNA, requires well preserved nucleic acid molecules which could be extremely difficult to isolate from fixed biological tissues. While Southern blot is currently not amenable to automation and produces considerable amounts of dilute radioactive waste, it is useful in studying viruses such as HPV since it can detect integration of the viral genome into the host genome, and may be used to test for specific HPV subtypes. [25] Compared to PCR, the Southern blot produces fewer false positives, but requires a much higher magnitude of DNA. [25] Both procedures are highly sensitive, detecting <0.1 copy of a given DNA sequence per cell. [25]

B.2. In Situ Hybridisation (ISH)

ISH is a technique that allows for the visualization of precise localised nucleic acid sequences within a histological section, by the application of a complementary strand of nucleic acid attached to a reporter molecule (e.g. radioactive isotopes, biotin, fluorescent dye

– FISH), provided that the nucleic acids are preserved adequately in the specimen. [34] Probes may be dsDNA probes, ssDNA probes, riboprobes, or synthetic oligonucleotides [34] Riboprobes may be used to localize and assess the degree of gene expression. [34]

ISH is a common method for HPV DNA detection in formalin fixed paraffin embedded (FFPE) sections, however, it is less sensitive compared to qRT-PCR (it cannot detect <10-50 viral copies per cell), and less specific for HPV DNA compared to Southern blot. [25, 31, 35] This is not an acceptable level of sensitivity since most HPV-positive OSCC cells harbor fewer than 50 HPV copies per cell. [35] Contrary to these findings, Stransky et al., used a HPV pan-specific DNA probe to recognize HPV subtypes 6, 11, 16, 18, 31, 33, 35, 45, 51 and 52 and found 98.7% agreement between PCR and ISH in their HNSCC samples. [36] It is considered that signals originating within the cell nuclei indicate HPV genome integration, but this is not necessarily true. [25] ISH requires relatively abundant nucleic acids for detection. In order to amplify the target and signal and increase its sensitivity, ISH has been combined with in-situ PCR to detect amplified mRNA as an indirect marker of gene expression. [37] The potential for error in HPV typing because of cross-hybridization and limitations such as difficulty in reproducibility and target localization lead to combining ISH with catalyzed signal amplification (CSA-ISH). [38] Compared to PCR-ISH, CSA-ISH is simpler and faster and has been shown to be more sensitive than ISH and is supposedly as sensitive as PCR, detecting one or two copies of HPV DNA. [35] However, optimization of this method is difficult and there is the possibility that background staining is misinterpreted as punctate HPV-positive staining. [35]

A new chromogenic RNA ISH assay, RNAscope® (Advanced Cell Diagnostics, Inc., Hayward, CA), has been utilized recently to detect E6/E7 mRNA of HR-HPV types on tissue microarrays, showing greater sensitivity compared to DNA ISH in detecting HPV in OPSCC and correlating strongly with p16. [39, 40] Bishop et al., [12] confirmed this stating it was the ideal detection method as it ratifies the presence of integrated and transcriptionally active virus, permits visualization of viral transcripts in tissues, and is technically feasible for routine testing in clinical laboratories. They argue that the transcription of viral mRNA provides a natural target amplification step that can improve viral detection in clinical samples and clarify the status of tumours that are p16 positive but HPV negative by DNA ISH. [12] They also found that HPV DNA ISH did not detect HPV DNA in 20% of cases that expressed mRNA E6/E7 transcripts. [12] However, Dreyer et al., [41] found that while it was a sensitive tool for HPV infection, it did not discriminate between E6/E7 transcripts and viral DNA based on two facts. One was that manufacturer's instructions included a 100°C heat treatment step which they suspected was not sufficient to denature viral DNA. Secondly, they observed two types of signals in positive cases, of which one type of signal did not completely disappear following RNase digestion. The signal that was retained was a similar pattern to what they obtained during DNA ISH.

Advantages of ISH include the ability to assay FFPE sections without further processing, the visualization of results on a standard pathology microscope, and the ability to determine whether the hybridization occurs in tumour tissue or in normal epithelial tissues.[25] The major disadvantage is the potential for error in HPV typing because of probe cross-hybridisation. [23]

B.3. Polymerase Chain Reaction (PCR) and Variants

PCR is the process whereby the complementary strand to a specific template DNA sequence is amplified exponentially by DNA polymerase. [42] Billions of copies of the target sequence are accumulated at the end of the PCR reaction. [42] In reverse transcription PCR (RT-PCR), sample RNA is first converted to complementary DNA (cDNA) using purified reverse transcriptase before the PCR reaction. [25, 42] PCR may be used to detect any HPV infection, using degenerate primers that amplify multiple HPV subtypes, or a single subtype of HPV may be used to confirm prior detection of the same, with up to 95% sensitivity. [25] Furthermore, RT-PCR assays for E6 and E7 transcripts may be more reliable for detection of oncogenic HPV infections. [43]

Both PCR and RT-PCR amplification are highly sensitive techniques owing to the exponential amplification of target sequences lying between two priming sequences. [25, 43] These techniques have the potential to detect a single copy of a target sequence within a given sample in theory. [25] However, in practice, this high sensitivity can lead to false positive results either through the inclusion of random HPV genomes (particularly problematic in laboratories which commonly study HPV) or by detection of HPV genomes within the investigated tissues, but that are not causative for the malignancy. [25] In a study by Lee et al., [43] the possibility of laboratory artifacts and the presence of environmental virions were ruled out by performing all amplifications in duplicate with the use of two different PCR assays. Size of the PCR product, the primer set, the spectrum of HPV subtypes amplified, reaction conditions and performance of the DNA polymerase used in the reaction are some of the factors that determine the sensitivity and specificity of PCR-based methods in detection of HPV. [23] The most widely used PCR assay to detect a spectrum of HPV types used a primer designed to detect a highly conserved region of L1 protein and therefore identifies all mucosal HPV types. [44] Although detection of a wide spectrum of HPV types has been preferred, using type-specific assays has the benefit of very high specificity and sensitivity. [23] Extrapolation back to the starting quantity of the target sequence in the sample can only be done during the exponential phase of the PCR reaction since inhibitors of the polymerase reaction (reagent limitation, accumulation of pyrophosphate molecules, and self-annealing of the accumulating product) in the sample leads to the cessation of the PCR reaction and the exponential amplification of the target sequence, resulting in a “plateau effect”, making the end point quantification of PCR products unreliable. [42] These limitations created the need for probe-based real-time quantitative PCR (qRT-PCR). [42]

The aim of qRT-PCR is to quantify the amplified PCR products (amplicons) in real-time, as the PCR reaction occurs. [45, 46] It uses a specially-designed ssDNA probe that hybridizes within the target DNA sequence. [45] One of the nucleotides is labelled with a fluorescent molecule and another nucleotide is labelled with a quencher molecule. [45] The latter rapidly absorbs any light emitted by the fluorescent molecule as long as it remains in close proximity. [45] Due to the exonuclease activity of DNA polymerase, this probe is disassembled during the PCR reaction cycle, and the fluorescent-labelled nucleotide is separated from the quencher-labelled nucleotide. [45] This allows for the fluorescent molecule to emit detectable light when stimulated. [45] Therefore, as the number of amplicons increase with each PCR cycle, the amount of emitted fluorescent energy also doubles, which can be monitored with a fluorometer during the reaction. [45] Therefore, the amount of specific DNA in the clinical sample is determined in reference to the round of PCR in which the amount of fluorescence first crosses the threshold of detection (fractional PCR cycle number; Ct). [45, 46] Frequently, reverse transcription is performed prior to qualitative PCR in order to convert RNA to cDNA. [45, 46] qRT-PCR significantly reduces the risk of false positives and is particularly useful for detecting transcriptionally active HPV – i.e. it is able to determine whether a HPV infection has resulted in the production of viral proteins and mRNA. [25, 31] It may also be used to assess the degree of viral genome integration. Integration leads to loss of expression of L1 and E2 genes. [25] Hence, samples that express E6 and E7 but not L1 and E2 genes, are thought to harbour integrated HPV, whereas if all four viral genes are expressed, the sample would be considered to harbour episomal HPV. [25] For these reasons, qRT-PCR of viral E6/E7 mRNA is now considered the "gold standard" for the detection of clinically significant HPV infections within tumour specimens. [40] Furthermore, automation of each step of qRT-PCR is a major benefit to researchers. [25] Nevertheless, the possibility of target degradation when fresh frozen tissue is unavailable represents a significant limitation of both qRT-PCR and RT-PCR. [25]

Nested PCR, a variant of PCR that is particularly useful in HPV detection, identifies the presence of HPV DNA from total genomic DNA using two different sets of degenerate primers known to detect multiple mucosotropic HPV genomes, thus increasing the specificity of DNA amplification by reducing background non-specific DNA amplification. [47-50] This technique was developed by Williamson and Rybicki [50] to eliminate the amplification of HPV non-specific DNA – the second set of primers amplify a 335 bp sequence contained within the 441 bp sequence which is part of a well-conserved portion of the L1 capsid protein gene. [49] The nested primers are used in a two-stage PCR reaction to obtain distinct HPV-specific DNA fragments suitable for direct sequencing, yielding a 5-fold higher sensitivity compared to single-step PCR [49, 50].

HPV Direct Flow CHIP is a newly developed test that identifies 18 high risk and 18 low risk HPV genotypes using direct PCR of [GP5+/GP6+]-based multiplex amplification from crude-cell extracts (therefore not requiring previous DNA extraction), automatic flow-through hybridization, and colorimetric detection. [51] The analytical sensitivity and specificity has been shown to be 100% by the 2011 WHO HPV LabNet Proficiency Study (manuscript in preparation). [51] The results of this method have been found to be comparable with Linear Array HPV Genotyping Test, CLART HPV2, and Digene Hybrid Capture 2 HPV DNA Test, however, it is yet to be compared against a gold standard reference method. [51]

B.4. Next Generation Sequencing (NGS)

NGS works by restriction digestion of sample DNA producing thousands of DNA fragments, or reverse transcription of sample RNA with recent advances allowing for direct RNA sequencing. [25] Thousands of these fragments are simultaneously sequenced rapidly, accurately, and comprehensively by NGS using high-throughput technology. [25, 52] Newer technologies aim to make the process even faster and more cost-effective, making it feasible to perform whole genome amplification (WGA) of a tumour in a few hours. [25, 53] Each commercial platform differs by the technology it uses to determine the nucleotide sequence. [25, 54] NGS has the potential to offer insight into somatic and genetic alterations in tumour genomes by providing the opportunity to compare the tumour sequence to germline, enabling personalized patient care. [54, 55] The differences between HPV-positive and HPV-negative OSCC calls for a refined tumour classification system, [55] and NGS is expected to contribute significantly to this end.

NGS is a highly sensitive assay requiring only a little input DNA and can detect variant DNA at very low frequencies. [25, 53] It is able to process tumour samples for HPV DNA, determine viral genome copy number, and identify co-infections with multiple viral genome subtypes or associations with alternative viral aetiologies. [25, 56, 57] Traditional methods require the use of both PCR and p16 IHC, while NGS provides multiple clinically significant data from heterogeneous tumour specimens in a single test, and FFPE samples may also be used. [57, 58] However, there are still some important considerations when using this assay, such as the preparation of sequencing libraries with molecular barcodes, methods to calculate diagnostic sensitivity, and the choice of suitable software and data processing solutions to obtain accurate results (e.g. HPV-QUEST). [58, 59] Furthermore, it is still expensive. [25] Nevertheless, NGS is on the brink of having a massive impact on clinical practice.

Nichols et al., [60] recently performed high throughput mutational analysis of 6 HNSCC cancer cell lines and found *TP53* mutations in all cell lines and *CDKN2A* mutations in all cell lines except one. NGS of HNSCC primary tumours have previously been performed in studies by Agrawal et al., [61] and Stransky et al., [36] both of which highlight mutations deactivating the *NOTCH1* receptor and a high incidence of *TP53* and pRb mutations in HPV-negative tumours. This was also confirmed in a more recent study with larger sample sizes and using paired-end sequencing of hybrid-captured DNA, reporting *TP53* mutations in 100% of HPV-negative samples (n=20). [62] This study also demonstrated mutations or copy number alterations (CNAs) in genes that activate the PI3K/AKT/mTOR pathway in HPV-positive HNSCC, with >60% HPV-positive tumours and 31% HPV-negative tumors demonstrating *PIK3CA* mutation and *PTEN* inactivation by mutation or gene copy loss. Despite the fact that CDKN2A product, p16, has been commonly considered as a HPV marker, CDKN2A alterations have been reported to be independent of HPV infection. [36] Lechner et al., report *CCND1* amplification and *CDKN2A/B* deletions in ~55% of HPV-negative OPSCC cases each. [62]

Appraisal of HPV Detection Methodologies

While there is no current standard for testing or interpretation of HPV detection assays, each having its strengths and limitations, p16 IHC and HPV-16 ISH are currently preferred for prognostication; these methods being used in clinical trials proving HPV to be an important prognostic factor in OPSCC tumours. [21] Bussu et al., [27] suggested detection of viral mRNA in fresh samples and DNA detection in FFPE samples as the standard. PCR demonstrates viral oncogene transcription but does not provide information about the viral load and the distribution of HPV DNA, nor is it able to indicate the specific site of viral integration in the genome. [22, 63, 64] Studies tend to use PCR to detect HPV DNA without specifying viral load. [22] Targeting HPV RNA has the advantage of evaluating the viral activity through HPV genome expression and is particularly useful in identifying clinically relevant HPV infection, however RNA is less stable than DNA and hence less available in most biological specimens.

Since PCR can detect extremely small fragments of DNA, its high sensitivity generates false positive results, through sample contamination or biologically insignificant infection. [7, 22, 25, 65, 66] Jordan et al., reported 14% of HPV DNA-positive tumours were negative for HPV E6/7 expression and had a very low viral load, with the literature quoting up to 50%

discrepancy, demonstrating that PCR alone cannot be relied on for classification of HPV status due to generation of false-positives [14, 21].

In comparison, qRT-PCR, which utilizes a third probe lying within the target sequence, significantly decreases the risk of false positives, and can detect RNA sequences at much lower concentrations. [25] The major limitation of both PCR and qRT-PCR is the risk of target degradation when fresh frozen tissue is unavailable. [25] ISH assays for HPV DNA and provides data on the presence of HPV in different cells, but has limited sensitivity for certain HPV genotypes, cannot demonstrate oncogene transcription, and also does not pinpoint the specific site of viral integration in the genome. [22, 63, 64] However, ISH can detect HPV-negative infected cells with low viral loads and show the distribution of HPV DNA within the tumour. [22, 64] p16 IHC and HPV16 ISH have excellent concordance but about 15% of results are p16 positive but HPV16 ISH negative, at least half of which were attributed to other HPV genotypes. [21] Bishop et al., [12] found up to 18% of all OPSCC cases to be p16 positive by IHC but HPV negative by DNA ISH (based on standard protocol at Johns Hopkins Hospital to evaluate all OPSCC cases with a combination of detection assays). They stated that the use of E6/E7 mRNA detection method by RNA ISH could reduce the number of such cases and found transcriptionally active HPV in 84% of p16-positive cases in which 1 or more of the HPV DNA probes (a broad spectrum cocktail of 18 HR-HPV genotypes) failed to detect HPV. [12] Jordan et al., also reported ~3% of OPSCC cases were p16 negative and HPV16 ISH positive but with HPV E6/7 expression, and were aetiologically associated with HPV. [21] The molecular pathways resulting in p16 overexpression in the absence of HPV expression, and the lack of p16 expression in the presence of HR-HPV E6/7 expression are not clear, and the clinical outcomes of patients displaying these discordant results are yet to be elucidated. [21] Jordan et al., [21] advise that approximately 17% to 19% of cases would be misclassified based on p16 IHC or HPV16 ISH alone, yielding numerous false positives and false negatives respectively. However, Bishop and colleagues suggest that p16 may be induced by nonviral mechanisms in a subset of p16-positive OPSCC, but concede that HPV detection solely based on p16 overexpression is useful for prognostication since p16 overexpression has been associated with improved patient outcomes in patients with OPSCC, independent of HPV status. [11, 12, 67]

A systematic review and meta-analysis of 124 studies by Petrick et al.,[68] found average HPV prevalence among oesophageal SCC cases to be 0.277 by PCR, 0.243 by ISH, 0.304 by IHC, 0.322 by L1 serology, and 0.176 by Southern blot, with the highest prevalence found in populations in regions of China with a high incidence of oesophageal SCC. This study highlights the impact of HPV detection method, continent, publication date, and study size on the results of individual studies accounting for the large variability. They also highlighted the need to account for background prevalence of HPV which also varies significantly between populations. Syrjanen et al., [69] found 30.6% of oesophageal SCC cases tested positive for HPV in their systematic review and meta-analysis, also reporting variation when stratifying for detection method.

A RNA-based real time, nucleic acid sequence-based amplification assay (NASBA) (PreTect HPV-Proofer; Nanochip, West-fjorden, Norway) that tests for HPV types 16, 18, 31, 33 and 45 has been shown to be more specific than HPV testing for DNA detection by PCR. [70] Gao et al., [31] compared a new qRT-PCR method for the expression profiling of E6 and E7 from 13 HR-HPV genotypes with HPV RNA ISH and concluded that qRT-PCR and ISH were both equally effective in determining HPV status, and were both highly sensitive and specific methods. However, the authors noted that ISH is not quantitative and requires positive and negative controls for appropriate staining of each case. [31] ISH, being slide based, is useful for small tissue samples which may not yield enough RNA for qRT-PCR. [31] The authors also found that HPV detection by qRT-PCR and p16 detection either by qRT-PCR or IHC led to equivalent results, however HPV DNA detection by ISH alone has a relatively low sensitivity. [31]

While many authors have studied detection of HPV in cancerous tissues, only a few have focused on optimizing the detection methods based on the interaction of HPV with the host in potentially malignant lesions. Klaes et al., [71] based their diagnostic method on the fact that viral DNA is usually kept as episomes in normal and potentially malignant tissues compared to cervical cancer where viral genome is integrated into the host chromosomes.

While PCR, ISH and IHC are currently used in combination to identify HPV DNA and RNA expression, NGS is now emerging as a strong contender in diagnostic technology. It is recommended that NGS be utilised to its full potential in sequencing HPV-positive OPSCC and oral epithelial dysplasia (OED) compared with controls to illuminate the molecular difference between HPV positive and negative OPSCC, saving time and attaining a diverse data set through a relatively simple procedure. Until the widespread uptake of NGS, HPV testing using a combination of laboratory methods is indicated to determine treatment protocols for patients with true HPV-positive OPSCC.

HPV-Positive HNSCC

While tobacco and alcohol exposure are established risk factors for HNSCC, a unique subset has developed which is often associated with HPV with many studies demonstrating a survival outcome advantage even in patients with nodal involvement. [11, 13, 72-75] Epidemiological studies have shown that these tumours occur more frequently in the oropharynx (especially lingual and palatine tonsils and base of the tongue), among younger patients, higher socioeconomic groups, and those exposed to more sexual partners and oral sex compared to HPV-negative HNSCC. [15, 75-79] The tumours related to tobacco and alcohol exposure appear to be declining while tonsillar and oropharyngeal tumours related to HPV seem to be on the rise. [75, 80-83] While HPV is not yet fully established as a causative factor of oropharyngeal epithelial dysplasia or OPSCC, the reported increased incidence of OPSCC is considered to be related to changing sexual patterns, namely orogenital contact which increases the rate of oral HPV transmission. [3, 7, 84] HPV might play an aetiological role in carcinogenesis of the oral cavity and might have a molecular mechanism similar to that found in cervical cancer. [85] It has been recently found that a history of cervical cancer increases the risk of oral cavity and oropharyngeal cancer development to over 6 times that of the general female population (relative risk of HNC development subsequent to cervical cancer was 6.7), further increasing the suspicion that the two cancers share similar aetiological factors. [86]

Based on the discussion of HPV detection methods, the reasons for inter-study variability in reported HPV prevalence is clear. Despite this, it has been established that transcriptionally active HR-HPV genotypes have been preferentially found in the oropharynx and that HPV-16 is the most prevalent subtype. [12, 87-90] Only a small subset of HNSCCs arising in the larynx, hypopharynx and oral cavity exhibited transcriptionally active E6/E7 mRNA, [91] although some recent studies have shown a subset of HPV-related tumours arising in the oral cavity. [5, 92, 93] It has been noted that up to 20% of sinonasal HNSCCs harbor HR-HPV. [90, 94, 95]

The predilection of HR-HPV for the oropharynx and tonsils could be related to the tonsillar microanatomy, making these regions prone to infection and early metastases. The surface of the tonsil is covered with epithelium-lined pits, called tonsillar crypts, that pass into the underlying lymphoid tissue. [96] Tonsillar epithelium originates from the mesoderm and ectoderm, with crypts that are populated by lymphocytes. [97] The palatine and lingual tonsils are lined with stratified squamous epithelium, also in the crypts. [97] The pharyngeal tonsils, however, are lined by ciliated, pseudostratified columnar epithelium, similar to that of the respiratory passages, have shallow infoldings called pleats instead of crypts, and tend to atrophy after childhood. [97, 98] The stratified squamous epithelium extends into the crypt for some distance but as they merge with the underlying lymphoid tissue, the epithelial cells assume a more basaloid appearance (i.e. high nuclear-to-cytoplasmic ratio, absence of cytoplasmic keratinization) with vesicular nuclei and loss of distinct cytoplasmic borders and intercellular bridges. [96, 99] It is considered that HPV-related OPSCCs arise from this crypt epithelium, particularly of the lingual and palatine tonsils, both of which lie within the oropharynx. [96] The preferential targeting possibly reflects the complex biological interactions between HPV and the specialized lympho-epithelium lining the tonsillar crypts, known as reticulated epithelium. [99]

Premalignant lesions arising in the oropharyngeal tonsillar crypts are difficult to identify accounting for compromised understanding of HPV associated oral potentially malignant lesions (OPML). [5] While tonsillar 'crypt dysplasia' should theoretically exist and be detectable, invasion and metastasis may occur at an early stage in tumour development since the tonsillar crypt epithelium contains numerous small blood vessels and has a discontinuous basement membrane. [5] It is highly possible for small occult stage T1 tumours to be associated with metastases to regional neck lymph nodes. [5] Therefore any "precursor" lesions may truly be invasive carcinomas. [5] HR-HPV in OED has been associated with a subset of severe epithelial dysplasia or carcinoma in situ by McCord et al.. [92] Syrjanen and colleagues reported an increased risk of HPV detection in oral cavity OPML and dysplasia relative to controls. [100] It has also been found that the presence of HPV-16 in OED and the occurrence of p16 (CDKN2A) methylation are associated. While both are associated with tissue transformation, it is as yet to be determined if these factors behave independently or synergistically with any impact on malignant transformation of OED. [101] A meta-analysis by Jayaprakash et al., [102] calculated the overall prevalence for HPV-16/18 in oropharyngeal epithelial dysplasia to be 24.5%, while the prevalence of HPV-16 alone in these cases was 24.4%. Compared to normal biopsies, HPV-16/18 were detected 3 times more in dysplastic lesions and invasive cancers. They also did not find any difference in HPV prevalence between dysplastic lesions and cancers, or between mild, moderate or severe dysplastic lesions. In contrast, Feller and Lemmer [7] did not find enough evidence to prove a causal association between HPV and the development or progression of oral leukoplakia.

A. Histopathology

HPV-related HNSCC has not been well characterized microscopically. Islands of squamous epithelial cells without keratinization, compared to conventional severe dysplasia, and invasive growth are features of this tumour. [5, 103] Cells typically lack maturation and display moderate to significant atypia with 'koilocytic' features. [5, 103, 104] HPV-related tumours have characteristic bowenoid histologic features (resembling Bowen's disease of skin) described as 'basaloid' with diffuse, full-thickness loss of squamous differentiation and a high proliferation index throughout the basal and suprabasal epithelial layers. [5, 92] Mitotic-figures and mitotic-like structures, multinucleated cells, dyskeratotic cells and apoptosis can be seen throughout the thickness of the epithelium. [5, 92, 93] Secondary morphologic features have been described by Westra [99] to include the presence of central necrosis with cystic change, tumour infiltrating lymphocytes, and basaloid features. He also adds that surface dysplasia and prominent stromal desmoplasia may also be absent. El-Mofty [105] describes some of the variants in histological presentation of HPV-related SCC.

B. Natural History

The HPV viral particle gains access into the epithelial basal cells (consisting of stem cells and transit-amplifying cells) through microabrasions of the epithelial tissue. [16] Infection of the continuously dividing stem cells, that replace the desquamating superficial layer cells, is necessary for maintenance of the infection. [16] The viral early genes are expressed while the keratinocyte is in the basal or parabasal layer, while the late genes are expressed as the keratinocyte reaches the upper spinous, stratified or cornified layers. [106] Persistent infection, which the host immune system has been incapable of clearing, has been deemed a causal factor for cervical carcinoma. [107]

HR-HPV E6 and E7 proteins are oncogenic proteins capable of inducing cell growth and transformation. [16, 19] E6 binds to p53 (a tumour suppressor protein) by ubiquitination forming a complex in conjunction with ubiquitin ligase (E6AP), leading to proteolytic degradation of p53 and consequent impaired apoptosis following DNA damage and cellular immortalization. [18, 108] E7 binds to and inactivates the retinoblastoma protein (pRb, also a tumour suppressor protein) which reduces binding to E2F, resulting in proliferation, malignant transformation, and cell cycle deregulation through S-phase entry. [18, 108] Destabilization of pRb also results in the upregulation of the p16 tumour suppressor protein (a cyclin-dependent kinase inhibitor located on gene *CDKN2A*), which inhibits the phosphorylation of the Rb-E2F complex. [31, 108] E7 also interacts with p21, inhibiting cyclins and subsequently restraining cell cycle arrest. [108] Further interactions with a number of other cell proteins (BAK, telomerase, cyclins A and E, WAF1, and KIP1) lead to cell immortalization and genome instability by deactivation of control and regulatory mechanisms of cell apoptosis. [8] Evidence continues to accumulate that HPV retains a sustained and critical role in cellular transformation. [7, 12, 18]

Based on the natural history of the virus, from viral infection, to viral persistence, to virus-induced malignant transformation, additional methods of HPV detection will continue to emerge (Figure 1). [12]

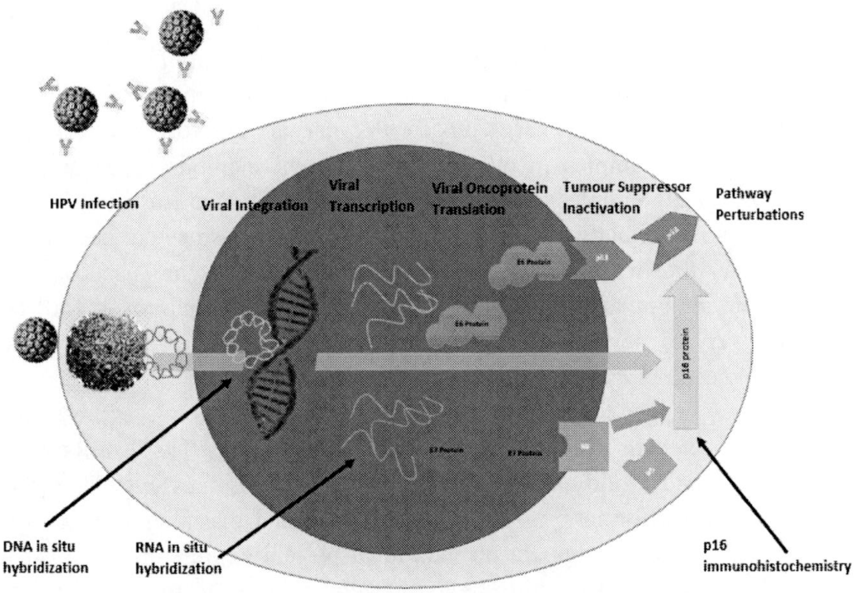

Figure 1. Based on the natural history of HPV in host cells, there are a number of methods to detect and confirm transcriptionally active (biologically relevant) HPV [Figure adapted from Bishop et al., [12].

C. miRs in HPV-Positive HNSCC

miRs are small, single-stranded RNA molecules that were first discovered in 1993, shown to influence the larval development of the nematode *Caenorhabditis elegans* by regulating translation through an antisense RNA-RNA interaction. [109-113] Although they are non-coding, they are considered to influence the expression of many protein coding genes in the human genome. [114] miRs are associated with mRNA translation and degradation, influencing organ development, cell differentiation, proliferation, apoptosis, and stress responses. [107-109, 115] Multiple miRs can target one mRNA, while one miR can influence mRNA transcripts of numerous genes, [114] implicating them in tumour development by modulation of cellular levels of specific oncogenes or tumour suppressor genes. [109, 116] Studying miR dysregulation in HPV-associated HNSCC can shed more light on the association between HPV and cellular change, and can also develop into a set of biomarkers for detection and diagnosis of these cancers.

Lajer et al., [108] identified a set of core miRs implicated in HPV pathogenesis in HPV-positive HNSCC, namely, miR-15a/miR-16/miR-195/miR-497 family, miR-143/miR-145, and the miR-106-363 cluster. Gao et al., [117] investigated the miR profile in HPV-positive OPSCC and found that five miRs were significantly correlated – miR-9, -223, -31, -18a, and -155. Wald et al., [118] studied the miR expression profile in HPV16-positive and HPV-negative HNSCC cell lines. miR-363, -33, and -497 were upregulated, while miR-155, -181a, -181b, -29a, -218, -222, -221, and -142-5p were downregulated. In a recent study, Hui et al,. [119] found upregulated miR-20b, -9, and -9* associated with HPV/p16 status in OPSCC. They also identified three candidate prognostic miR sets significantly associated with overall survival (miR-107, -151, -492), disease-free survival (miR-20b, -107, -151, -182, -361), and distant metastasis (miR-151, -152, -324-5p, -361, -492), independent of p16 status. [119]

It is evident that the results of most of these studies are conflicting and inconsistent, and no clear pattern has emerged. [120] Reasons for this may be due to the use of cell lines in some studies, and FFPE samples in others, with different methods used for pathological staging and grading. [120] Samples may also be from varying anatomical sites. [120].

Cell lines cannot recapitulate miR profiling of solid tumours since culture conditions and clonal selection may drastically alter miR expression, [120] but are used since they are inexpensive, easy to manipulate, and easily available for research purposes. [60] Moreover, the ongoing discovery of new miRs compels continued profiling in search of appropriate diagnostic and prognostic biomarkers. [120]

There are large changes in miR expression compared to mRNA expression between normal cells and cancer cells thus aiding detection of differences. [121] miRs are also less prone to degradation and modification in FFPE tissue samples thus expediently supplying significant retrospective information. [121] It has been found that alterations in single miR expression have only a modest impact on individual protein expression. [122, 123] Global miR screening is therefore considered to be more useful in order to study collective changes in miR expression, since it is more likely that miRs work cooperatively *in vivo* to physiologically regulate proteins. [124] In accordance with this, Lajer et al., [108] observed that deregulation of a single miR implicates the collective action of a cluster of miRs or a whole miR family, consequently influencing multiple proteins in a complex manner.

D. HPV-Positive HNSCC and the Epigenome

Promoter hypermethylation is a well-documented mechanism for tumour-specific alteration of suppressor gene activity in human malignancy, including HNSCC. [125] However, there are limited studies attending to the difference in epigenetic alteration in HPV-positive and HPV-negative HNSCC. [126] The existing data is based on changes in promoter methylation of a limited number of candidate genes selected based on functional relevance in several human malignancies. [126] Sartor et al., [127] found higher overall DNA methylation in HPV-positive compared to HPV-negative cell lines, which is also consistent with findings by Richards et al., [128] who used primary tumour samples. Biron et al., [129] found that p16-positive and p16-negative OPSCCs have distinct epigenetic profiles representing broad gene expression differences between these tumours having found differences in histone levels. Nevertheless, due to the possible differences in DNA methylation patterns between cell lines and tumour samples, critical validation in larger HNSCC tumour sample sets is required. [126]

E. Prognosis

The presence of oncogenic HPV DNA in HNSCC is considered to be a good prognostic indicator (lower mortality rate, [74] lower risk of recurrence, [74, 130] better response to chemotherapy, [131] and improved progression-free survival [13, 130]), [125, 132] however, the reason for this is unknown. [83, 133-135] Two recent high-throughput sequencing studies found more mutations in HPV-negative HNSCC than HPV-positive HNSCC. [61, 136] Additionally, while TP53 mutations are the most common mutation in HNSCC, it is a rare occurrence in HPV-positive tumours, indicating a distinct biological mechanism of tumorigenesis. [61, 62, 136] p16 overexpression has been associated with improved patient outcomes in patients with OPSCCs, independent of HPV status. [11, 12, 67] In contrast, while Nygård et al., [137] demonstrated a population level increased survival in HPV-positive OPSCCs in the period 1981-2007 in Norway, they could not attribute this trend to changes in treatment, cancer registration or screening, but considered it to be due to an increased prevalence of HPV-positive tumours.

Conversely, one study conducted in Taiwan found that patients with advanced HPV-positive OSCC undergoing radical surgery and radiation-based adjuvant therapy did not have a lower risk of disease relapse or better survival, compared with case-matched HPV-negative OSCC patients. [43] The authors further found that distant metastases was 3 times as likely to occur in advanced HPV-16-positive OSCC patients, and were 2-3 times more likely to die earlier compared to HPV-negative patients, [43] which could be due to the blurred junction between the reticulated epithelium in the tonsillar crypt and the underlying lymphoid stroma and its porous nature. Duray et al., [138] found a decreased 5-year survival rate in Belgian patients with HR-HPV-positive OSCC compared with low risk HPV-positive OSCC and HPV-negative OSCC. Furthermore, there is some evidence that concomitant tobacco users have worse outcomes and should be classified as "intermediate risk" between non-smoking HPV-positive cases and HPV-negative cases. [136]

While genomic changes exist in both HPV-positive and HPV-negative tumours, the total amount of chromosomal alterations and amplifications are less in the former subset of HNSCC, which could also contribute to the improved clinical outcome of these cases. [126] This finding is consistent with the assumption that due to the inactivation of p53 and pRb by viral proteins, fewer genetic alterations are required to reach a malignant phenotype. [126] There are, however, specific HPV-related genetic modifications, some of which are associated with improved survival, for example, 16q loss and 18q12.1 – 23 gain in HPV-positive OPSCC. [139-143]

F. Treatment

Primary treatment for patients with HNSCC is largely determined by the clinical stage at diagnosis. [144] The NCCN guidelines for management of oropharyngeal cancer stipulates that HPV testing should not guide treatment and the results should not influence management decisions, but should be used for its prognostic value and also because prior HPV infection is related to the development of a significant proportion of OPSCCs. [15] These guidelines recommend definitive radiation therapy for OPSCC (T1-2, N0-1) as first line treatment. [15] Transoral or open resection of primary tumour with or without ipsilateral or bilateral neck dissection should be considered for more involved cases. [15] As the staging worsens, concurrent systemic therapy with radiotherapy (RT) should be considered, where the preferred agent is cisplatin. [15] Enrollment in multimodality clinical trials should also be considered. [15] Salvage surgery is recommended for managing residual or recurrent disease. [15] Induction chemotherapy followed by RT or chemoradiation is suggested for locally or regional advanced cases, but most panel members prefer concurrent systemic therapy with

RT. [15] Simply put, the challenges associated with appropriate patient selection and management of treatment-related toxicities with induction chemotherapy make it an unpopular choice, and it is recommended that it should only be done in centers with expertise in these regimens. [15] Residual toxicity from induction chemotherapy may also complicate the subsequent delivery of definitive RT or chemotherapy/RT. [15]

Concomitant administration of cisplatin chemotherapy and RT reduces the risk of loco-regional recurrence and death in patients with HNSCC. [145] Palliative platinum-based chemotherapy (e.g. cisplatin and paclitaxel) is the standard of care for recurrent or metastatic disease. [144] Cetuximab, a monoclonal antibody to the epidermal growth factor (EGFR), is an alternative to cisplatin for chemoradiotherapy, [146] which also has improved survival when administered with palliative chemotherapy. [147]

Currently, while tumour HPV status is routinely used as a stratification factor or eligibility criteria for clinical trials involving OPSCC, HPV testing results do not affect the standard of care for patients with OPSCC outside of the context of a clinical trial, unless investigating cancers of unknown or occult primary, where HPV positive status may help to define radiation fields being investigated. [15, 144]

H. Radiotherapy in HPV-Positive HNSCC

It has been demonstrated that HPV-positive HNSCC cells are intrinsically less sensitive to cisplatin treatment in vitro compared to HPV-negative cell lines, but the responses to cetuximab and radiation are similar with comparable migratory capacities. [10] Hence, based on this in vitro study by Nagel et al., the use of cisplatin in the treatment of patients with HPV-positive HNSCC should be re-evaluated. [10] Lastly, the improved prognosis of HPV-positive HNSCC cannot be easily explained by an intrinsic sensitivity to chemoradiation, however, considering the reported improved prognosis of such tumours, the authors continue to recommend deintensified treatment protocols, tested in clinical trials. [10] The NCCN Panel found the available data on deintensified treatment protocols to be limited, and do not recommend this approach, [15] but they do recommend the use of cisplatin. [15]

Tang et al., [148] have shown that HNSCC cancer stem cells (CSC) are more resistant to cisplatin than non-CSC, suggesting that cisplatin may aid in tumour shrinkage but is less effective in CSC eradication, leaving behind this potent group of cancer cells. The authors also found that HPV status did not have an impact on the proportion of CSCs present in HNSCC or their sensitivity to cisplatin therapy, and suggested immune-regulated mechanisms may be responsible for favourable outcomes in HPV-positive HNSCC patients. [148]

Vermeer et al., [149] demonstrated that clearance of HPV-positive OPSCC during treatment with radiation and chemotherapy required an immune response, which was likely to be responsible for the observed improved clinical outcomes. They further described a radiation-induced change in tumour surface protein expression, allowing the body to recognize and aid in immune-mediated tumour clearance – decreased surface expression of CD47, a self-marker. [149] While CD47 is usually overexpressed in HNSCC, radiation induced a decrease in CD47 in a dose-dependent manner, whereas the protein levels on adjacent, normal tissues remained unaffected. [149] Cessation of sublethal radiation exposure was found to result in restoration of tumour cell CD47 protein levels. [149] Reduction in tumour cell CD47 expression increased phagocytosis of these cells by dendritic cells, leading to increased IFN-gamma and granzyme production from mixed lymphoctyes. [149] Lastly, the authors also found that decreasing tumour cell CD47 in combination with standard radiation and chemotherapy resulted in improved immune-mediated tumour clearance in vivo. [149] These findings suggest that decreasing CD47 specifically on tumour cells may be a good therapeutic target for HPV related disease. [149]

Conclusion

HPV is an emerging aetiological factor for HNSCC. HPV-positive HNSCC is thought to arise predominantly in the oropharynx. The natural history of HPV in infected cells and interaction with cellular machinery suggests its role in carcinogenesis and tissue transformation. The resulting effect of these interactions is one reason for the numerous HPV detection methods available today. High throughput sequencing, HPV E6/E7 mRNA ISH and qRT-PCR are detection methods to be used to detect transcriptionally active HPV. p16 IHC is useful for prognostication. There are some distinct features of HPV-positive HNSCC, however laboratory methods are still required to determine true infection and transcriptional activity. While these tumours are generally considered to be associated with improved patient prognosis compared to HPV-negative HNSCC, nodal involvement and distant metastases can occur in the early stages of tumour development which can still negatively impact 5-year survival rates. Furthermore, these tumours tend to affect the epithelium at the base of tonsillar crypts which is a difficult if not impossible part of the anatomy to monitor and assess for premalignant changes. Hence diagnosed cases may be much further along in terms of staging than may be clinically (visibly) apparent. HNSCC of unknown primary or occult primary should raise suspicion of the primary tumour being in these locations. Studying miR and epigenetic changes can aid in early detection and diagnosis of suspected cases. Current treatment protocols recommend definitive RT increasing to concurrent systemic therapy/RT with neck dissection. Induction chemotherapy is not recommended. The effects of cetuximab compared to cisplatin should be considered in these cases.

Conflict of Interest Statement

The authors have no conflict of interest to declare in relation to the work presented in this chapter.

References

[1] Warnakulasuriya S. Global epidemiology of oral and oropharyngeal cancer. *Oral. Oncol.* 2009;45:309-316.

[2] Barnes L, Eveson JW, Reichart P, Sidransky D, eds. World Health Organization classification of tumours pathology and genetics of head and neck tumours. Lyon: IARC Press, 2005.

[3] Farah CS, Simanovic B, Dost F. Oral cancer in Australia 1982-2008: a growing need for opportunistic screening and prevention. *Aust. Dent. J.* 2014;59:349-359.

[4] Warnakulasuriya S. Living with oral cancer: Epidemiology with particular reference to prevalence and life-style changes that influence survival. *Oral. Oncology* 2010;46:407-410.

[5] Chernock RD, Nussenbaum B, Thorstad WL, et al., Extensive HPV-related carcinoma in situ of the upper aerodigestive tract with 'nonkeratinizing' histologic features. *Head Neck Pathol.* 2014;8:322-328.

[6] Zygogianni AG, Kyrgias G, Karakitsos P, et al., Oral squamous cell cancer: early detection and the role of alcohol and smoking. *Head Neck Oncol.* 2011;3:2.

[7] Feller L, Lemmer J. Oral leukoplakia as it relates to HPV infection: A review. *Int. J. Dent.* 2012;2012:1-7.

[8] Kansy K, Thiele O, Freier K. The role of human papillomavirus in oral squamous cell carcinoma: myth and reality. *Oral Maxillofac. Surg.* 2012;18:165-172.

[9] Chen KM, Stephen JK, Ghanem T, et al., Human papilloma virus prevalence in a multiethnic screening population. *Otolaryngol. Head Neck Surg.* 2013;148:436-442.

[10] Galm O, Herman JG, Baylin SB. The fundamental role of epigenetics in hematopoietic malignancies. *Blood Reviews* 2006;20:1-13.

[11] Ang KK, Harris J, Wheeler R, et al., Human Papillomavirus and Survival of Patients with Oropharyngeal Cancer. *New England Journal of Medicine* 2010;363:24-35.

[12] Bishop JA, Ma XJ, Wang H, et al., Detection of transcriptionally active high-risk HPV in patients with head and neck squamous cell carcinoma as visualized by a novel E6/E7 mRNA in situ hybridization method. *Am. J. Surg. Pathol.* 2012;36:1874-1882.

[13] Fakhry C, Westra WH, Cmelak SLA, et al., Improved survival of patients with human papillomavirus-positive head and neck squamous cell carcinoma in a prospective clinical trial. *J. Natl. Cancer Inst.* 2008;100:261-269.

[14] Weinberger PM, Yu Z, Haffty BG, et al., Molecular classification identifies a subset of human papillomavirus-associated oropharyngeal cancers with favorable prognosis. *J. Clin. Oncol.* 2006;24:736-747.

[15] Pfister DG, Spencer S. National comprehensive cancer network clinical practice guidelines in oncology 2014. Head and neck cancers. Version 2.2014. Washington, PA: National comprehensive cancer network, 2014. URL: 'http://www.nccn.org /professionals/physician_gls/pdf/head-and-neck.pdf'. Accessed October 2014.

[16] Conway MJ, Meyers C. Replication and assembly of human papillomaviruses. *J. Dent. Res.* 2009;88:307-317.

[17] Vidal L, Gillison ML. Human papillomavirus in HNSCC: recognition of a distinct disease type. *Hematol. Oncol. Clin. North Am.* 2008;22:1125-1142.

[18] Alibek K, Kakpenova A, Baiken Y. Role of infectious agents in the carcinogenesis of brain and head and neck cancers. *Infect Agent Cancer* 2013;8:7.

[19] Tezal M. Interaction between chronic inflammation and oral HPV infection in the etiology of head and neck cancers. *Int. J. Otolaryngol.* 2012;2012:1-9.

[20] Robinson M, Schache A, Sloan P, Thavaraj S. HPV specific testing: a requirement for oropharyngeal squamous cell carcinoma patients. *Head Neck Pathol.* 2012;6 Suppl 1:S83-90.

[21] Jordan RC, Lingen MW, Perez-Ordonez B, et al., Validation of methods for oropharyngeal cancer HPV status determination in US cooperative group trials. *Am. J. Surg. Pathol.* 2012;36:945-954.

[22] Feller L, Wood NH, Khammissa RA, Lemmer J. Human papillomavirus-mediated carcinogenesis and HPV-associated oral and oropharyngeal squamous cell carcinoma. Part 2: Human papillomavirus associated oral and oropharyngeal squamous cell carcinoma. *Head Face Med.* 2010;6:15.

[23] Villa LL, Denny L. Methods for detection of HPV infection and its clinical utility. *Int. J. Gynaecol. Obstet.* 2006;94:S71-S80.

[24] Wang HK, Duffy AA, Broker TR, Chow LT. Robust production and passaging of infectious HPV in squamous epithelium of primary human keratinocytes. *Genes Dev.* 2009;23:181-194.

[25] Kimple AJ, Torres AD, Yang RZ, Kimple RJ. HPV-associated head and neck cancer: molecular and nano-scale markers for prognosis and therapeutic stratification. *Sensors (Basel)* 2012;12:5159-5169.

[26] Lingen MW, Xiao W, Schmitt A, et al., Low etiologic fraction for high-risk human papillomavirus in oral cavity squamous cell carcinomas. *Oral. Oncol.* 2013;49:1-8.

[27] Bussu F, Sali M, Gallus R, et al., HPV infection in squamous cell carcinomas arising from different mucosal sites of the head and neck region. Is p16 immunohistochemistry a reliable surrogate marker? *Br. J. Cancer* 2013;108:1157-1162.

[28] Poling JS, Ma XJ, Bui S, et al., Human papillomavirus (HPV) status of non-tobacco related squamous cell carcinomas of the lateral tongue. *Oral. Oncology* 2014.

[29] Shi W, Kato H, Perez-Ordonez B, et al., Comparative prognostic value of HPV16 E6 mRNA compared with in situ hybridization for human oropharyngeal squamous carcinoma. *J. Clin. Oncol.* 2009;27:6213-6221.

[30] Friedrich RE, Sperber C, Jakel T, Roser K, Loning T. Basaloid lesions of oral squamous epithelial cells and their association with HPV infection and P16 expression. *Anticancer Res.* 2010;30:1605-1612.

[31] Gao G, Chernock RD, Gay HA, et al., A novel RT-PCR method for quantification of human papillomavirus transcripts in archived tissues and its application in oropharyngeal cancer prognosis. *Int. J. Cancer* 2013;132:882-890.

[32] Wang W, Sima N, Kong D, et al., Selective targeting of HPV-16 E6/E7 in cervical cancer cells with a potent oncolytic adenovirus and its enhanced effect with radiotherapy in vitro and vivo. *Cancer Lett.* 2010;291:67-75.

[33] Suchankova A, Ritterova L, Krcmar M, et al., Comparison of ELISA and western blotting for human papillomavirus type 16 E7 antibody determination. *J. Gen. Virol.* 1991;72:2577-2581.

[34] NCBI probe - reagents for functional genomics. In situ hybridisation. Bethesda MD, USA. URL: 'http://www.ncbi.nlm.nih.gov/projects/ genome/probe/doc/TechISH.shtml'. Accessed May 2013.

[35] Acay R, Rezende N, Fontes A, Aburad A, Nunes F, Sousa S. Human papillomavirus as a risk factor in oral carcinogenesis: a study using in situ hybridization with signal amplification. *Oral. Microbiol. Immunol.* 2008;23:271-274.

[36] Stransky N, Egloff AM, Tward AD, et al., The mutational landscape of head and neck squamous cell carcinoma. *Science* 2011;333:1157-1160.

[37] Stoler MH, Wolinsky SM, Whitbeck A, Broker TR, Chow LT. Differentiation-linked human papillomavirus types 6 and 11 transcription in genital condylomata revealed by in situ hybridization with message-specific RNA probes. *Virology* 1989;172:331-340.

[38] Yokomori H, Oda M, Yasogawa Y, Nishi Y, Ishii H. Signal detection of endothelin receptor subtypes in human cirrhotic liver by a new in situ hybridization method. *Med. Electron Microsc.* 2000;33:207-216.

[39] Ukpo OC, Flanagan JJ, Ma XJ, Luo Y, Thorstad WL, Lewis JS, Jr. High-risk human papillomavirus E6/E7 mRNA detection by a novel in situ hybridization assay strongly correlates with p16 expression and patient outcomes in oropharyngeal squamous cell carcinoma. *Am. J. Surg. Pathol.* 2011;35:1343-1350.

[40] Venuti A, Paolini F. HPV detection methods in head and neck cancer. *Head Neck Pathol.* 2012;6 Suppl 1:S63-74.

[41] Dreyer JH, Hauck F, Oliveira-Silva M, Barros MH, Niedobitek G. Detection of HPV infection in head and neck squamous cell carcinoma: a practical proposal. *Virchows Arch.* 2013;462:381-389.

[42] NCBI probe - reagents for functional genomics. PCR. Bethesda MD, USA. URL: 'http://www.ncbi.nlm.nih.gov/projects/genome/probe/ doc/TechPCR.shtml'. Accessed May 2013.

[43] Lee LA, Huang CG, Liao CT, et al., Human papillomavirus-16 infection in advanced oral cavity cancer patients is related to an increased risk of distant metastases and poor survival. *PLoS One* 2012;7:1-11.

[44] Jacobs MV, Snijders PJ, Voorhorst FJ, et al., Reliable high risk HPV DNA testing by polymerase chain reaction: an intermethod and intramethod comparison. *J. Clin. Pathol.* 1999;52:498-503.

[45] Open Michigan. Laboratory methods for clinical microbiology. University of Michigan. Ann Arbor MI, USA. URL: 'http://open.umich.edu/education/med/oernetwork/med /microbiology/clinical-microbio-lab/2009'. Accessed May 2013.

[46] NCBI probe - reagents for functional genomics. Real-time qRT-PCR. Bethesda MD, USA. URL: 'http://www.ncbi.nlm.nih.gov/projects/ genome/probe/doc/TechQPCR. shtml'. Accessed May 2013.

[47] Kimple RJ, Harari PM, Torres AD, et al., Development and characterization of HPV-positive and HPV-negative head and neck squamous cell carcinoma tumorgrafts. *Clin. Cancer Res.* 2013;19:855-864.

[48] Snijders PJF, Vandenbrule AJC, Schrijnemakers HFJ, Snow G, Meijer C, Walboomers JMM. The use of general primers in the polymerase chain-reaction permits the detection of a broad-spectrum of human papillomavirus genotypes. *J. Gen. Virol.* 1990;71:173-181.

[49] Kay P, Meehan K, Williamson A-L. The use of nested polymerase chain reaction and restriction fragment length polymorphism for the detection and typing of mucosal human papillomaviruses in samples containing low copy numbers of viral DNA. *J. Virol. Methods* 2002;105:159-170.

[50] Williamson AL, Rybicki EP. Detection of genital human papillomaviruses by polymerase chain reaction amplification with degenerate nested primers. *J. Med. Virol.* 1991;33:165-171.

[51] Herraez-Hernandez E, Alvarez-Perez M, Navarro-Bustos G, et al., HPV Direct Flow CHIP: A new human papillomavirus genotyping method based on direct PCR from crude-cell extracts. *J. Virol. Methods* 2013;193:9-17.

[52] Metzker ML. Sequencing technologies - the next generation. *Nat. Rev. Genet* 2010;11:31-46.

[53] Elsharawy A, Warner J, Olson J, et al., Accurate variant detection across non-amplified and whole genome amplified DNA using targeted next generation sequencing. *BMC Genomics* 2012;13:500.

[54] Jessri M, Farah CS. Next generation sequencing and its application in deciphering head and neck cancer. *Oral. Oncol.* 2014; 50:247-253 .

[55] Jessri M, Farah CS. Harnessing massively parallel sequencing in personalized head and neck oncology. *J. Dent Res.* 2014; 93:437-444.

[56] Barzon L, Militello V, Lavezzo E, et al., Human papillomavirus genotyping by 454 next generation sequencing technology. *J. Clin. Virol.* 2011;52:93-97.

[57] Conway C, Chalkley R, High A, et al., Next-generation sequencing for simultaneous determination of human papillomavirus load, subtype, and associated genomic copy number changes in tumors. *J. Mol. Diagn* 2012;14:104-111.

[58] Kohlmann A, Grossmann V, Haferlach T. Integration of next-generation sequencing into clinical practice: are we there yet? *Semin. Oncol.* 2012;39:26-36.

[59] Yin L, Yao J, Gardner BP, Chang K, Yu F, Goodenow MM. HPV-QUEST: A highly customized system for automated HPV sequence analysis capable of processing Next Generation sequencing data set. *Bioinformation* 2012;8:388-390.

[60] Nichols AC, Yoo J, Palma DA, et al., Frequent mutations in TP53 and CDKN2A found by next-generation sequencing of head and neck cancer cell lines. *Arch. Otolaryngol. Head Neck Surg.* 2012;138:732-739.

[61] Agrawal N, Frederick MJ, Pickering CR, et al., Exome sequencing of head and neck squamous cell carcinoma reveals inactivating mutations in NOTCH1. *Science* 2011;333:1154-1157.

[62] Lechner M, Frampton GM, Fenton T, et al., Targeted next-generation sequencing of head and neck squamous cell carcinoma identifies novel genetic alterations in HPV+ and HPV- tumors. *Genome Med.* 2013;5:49.

[63] Gillison ML. Human papillomavirus and prognosis of oropharyngeal squamous cell carcinoma: implications for clinical research in head and neck cancers. *J. Clin. Oncol.* 2006;24:5623-5625.

[64] Miller CS, Zeuss MS, White DK. Detection of HPV DNA in oral carcinoma using polymerase chain reaction together with in situ hybridization. *Oral. Surg. Oral. Med. Oral. Pathol.* 1994;77:480-486.

[65] Ha PK, Califano JA. The role of human papillomavirus in oral carcinogenesis. *Crit. Rev. Oral. Biol. Med.* 2004;15:188-196.

[66] Hennessey PT, Westra WH, Califano JA. Human papillomavirus and head and neck squamous cell carcinoma: recent evidence and clinical implications. *J. Dent. Res.* 2009;88:300-306.

[67] Lewis JS, Jr., Thorstad WL, Chernock RD, et al., p16 positive oropharyngeal squamous cell carcinoma: an entity with a favorable prognosis regardless of tumor HPV status. *American Journal of Surgical Pathology* 2010;34:1088-1096.

[68] Petrick JL, Wyss AB, Butler AM, et al., Prevalence of human papillomavirus among oesophageal squamous cell carcinoma cases: systematic review and meta-analysis. *Br. J. Cancer* 2014;110:2369-2377.

[69] Syrjanen K. Geographic origin is a significant determinant of human papillomavirus prevalence in oesophageal squamous cell carcinoma: systematic review and meta-analysis. *Scand. J. Infect Dis.* 2013;45:1-18.

[70] Molden T, Kraus I, Karlsen F, Skomedal H, Nygard JF, Hagmar B. Comparison of human papillomavirus messenger RNA and DNA detection: a cross-sectional study of 4,136 women >30 years of age with a 2-year follow-up of high-grade squamous intraepithelial lesion. *Cancer Epidemiol. Biomarkers Prev.* 2005;14:367-372.

[71] Klaes R, Woerner SM, Ridder R, et al., Detection of high-risk cervical intraepithelial neoplasia and cervical cancer by amplification of transcripts derived from integrated papillomavirus oncogenes. *Cancer Res.* 1999;59:6132-6136.

[72] Chernock RD, El-Mofty SK, Thorstad WL, Parvin CA, Lewis JS, Jr. HPV-related nonkeratinizing squamous cell carcinoma of the oropharynx: utility of microscopic features in predicting patient outcome. *Head and neck pathology* 2009;3:186-194.

[73] Gillison ML, Koch WM, Capone RB, et al., Evidence for a causal association between human papillomavirus and a subset of head and neck cancers. *Journal of the National Cancer Institute* 2000;92:709-720.

[74] Ragin CCR, Taioli E. Survival of squamous cell carcinoma of the head and neck in relation to human papillomavirus infection: Review and meta-analysis. *Int. J. Cancer* 2007;121:1813-1820.

[75] Thomas J, Primeaux T. Is p16 immunohistochemistry a more cost-effective method for identification of human papilloma virus-associated head and neck squamous cell carcinoma? *Ann. Diagn Pathol.* 2012;16:91-99.

[76] El-Mofty SK, Lu DW. Prevalence of human papillomavirus type 16 DNA in squamous cell carcinoma of the palatine tonsil, and not the oral cavity, in young patients - A distinct clinicopathologic and molecular disease entity. *American Journal of Surgical Pathology* 2003;27:1463-1470.

[77] Gillison ML, D'Souza G, Westra W, et al., Distinct risk factor profiles for human papillomavirus type 16-positive and human papillomavirus type 16-negative head and neck cancers. *J. Natl. Cancer Inst.* 2008;100:407-420.

[78] Joseph AW, D'Souza G. Epidemiology of human papillomavirus-related head and neck cancer. *Otolaryngol. Clin. North Am.* 2012;45:739-764.

[79] Smith EM, Ritchie JM, Summersgill KF, et al., Age, sexual behavior and human papillomavirus infection in oral cavity and oropharyngeal cancers. *International Journal of Cancer* 2004;108:766-772.

[80] Ernster JA, Sciotto CG, O'Brien MM, et al., Rising incidence of oropharyngeal cancer and the role of oncogenic human Papilloma virus. *Laryngoscope* 2007;117:2115-2128.

[81] Hammarstedt L, Lindquist D, Dahlstrand H, et al., Human papillomavirus as a risk factor for the increase in incidence of tonsillar cancer. *International Journal of Cancer* 2006;119:2620-2623.

[82] Westra WH. The changing face of head and neck cancer in the 21st century: the impact of HPV on the epidemiology and pathology of oral cancer. *Head and neck pathology* 2009;3:78-81.

[83] Chaturvedi AK. Epidemiology and clinical aspects of HPV in head and neck cancers. *Head Neck Pathol* 2012;6 S16-S24.

[84] Heck JE, Berthiller J, Vaccarella S, et al., Sexual behaviours and the risk of head and neck cancers: a pooled analysis in the International Head and Neck Cancer Epidemiology (INHANCE) consortium. *Int. J. Epidemiol.* 2010;39:166-181.

[85] Angiero F, Gatta LB, Seramondi R, et al., Frequency and role of HPV in the progression of epithelial dysplasia to oral cancer. *Anticancer Res.* 2010;30:3435-3440.

[86] Dost F, Ford PJ, Farah CS. Heightened risk of second primary carcinoma of the head and neck following cervical neoplasia. *Head Neck* 2014;36:1132-1137.

[87] Begum S, Cao DF, Gillison M, Zahurak M, Westra WH. Tissue distribution of human papillomavirus 16 DNA integration in patients with tonsillar carcinoma. *Clinical Cancer Research* 2005;11:5694-5699.

[88] Singhi AD, Westra WH. Comparison of Human Papillomavirus In Situ Hybridization and p16 Immunohistochemistry in the Detection of Human Papillomavirus-Associated Head and Neck Cancer Based on a Prospective Clinical Experience. *Cancer* 2010;116:2166-2173.

[89] Chernock RD, Wang X, Gao G, et al., Detection and significance of human papillomavirus, CDKN2A(p16) and CDKN1A(p21) expression in squamous cell carcinoma of the larynx. Mod Pathol 2013;26:223-231.

[90] Syrjanen S. Human papillomavirus (HPV) in head and neck cancer. *J. Clin. Virol.* 2005;32 Suppl 1:S59-66.

[91] Lewis JS, Jr., Ukpo OC, Ma XJ, et al., Transcriptionally-active high-risk human papillomavirus is rare in oral cavity and laryngeal/hypopharyngeal squamous cell carcinomas--a tissue microarray study utilizing E6/E7 mRNA in situ hybridization. *Histopathology* 2012;60:982-991.

[92] McCord C, Xu J, Xu W, et al., Association of high-risk human papillomavirus infection with oral epithelial dysplasia. *Oral Surg Oral Med. Oral. Pathol. Oral. Radiol.* 2013;115:541-549.

[93] Woo SB, Cashman EC, Lerman MA. Human papillomavirus-associated oral intraepithelial neoplasia. *Mod. Pathol.* 2013;26:1288-1297.

[94] Bishop JA, Guo TW, Smith DF, et al., Human papillomavirus-related carcinomas of the sinonasal tract. *Am. J. Surg. Pathol.* 2013;37:185-192.

[95] El-Mofty SK, Lu DW. Prevalence of high-risk human papillomavirus DNA in nonkeratinizing (cylindrical cell) carcinoma of the sinonasal tract: a distinct clinicopathologic and molecular disease entity. *Am. J. Surg. Pathol.* 2005;29:1367-1372.

[96] Mills SE. Larynx and pharynx. In: Mills SE, ed. Histology for pathologists. 4th edn. *Wolters Kluwer/Lippincott Williams & Wilkins Health,* 2012:462-475.

[97] Syrjanen S. HPV infections and tonsillar carcinoma. *J. Clin. Pathol.* 2004;57:449-455.

[98] Gartner LP, Hiatt JL. Lymphoid (immune) system. In: Gartner LP, ed. Color textbook of histology. 3rd edn. Saunders/Elsevier, 2007:273-301.

[99] Westra WH. The morphologic profile of HPV-related head and neck squamous carcinoma: implications for diagnosis, prognosis, and clinical management. *Head Neck Pathol.* 2012;6 Suppl 1:S48-54.

[100] Syrjanen S, Lodi G, von Bultzingslowen I, et al., Human papillomaviruses in oral carcinoma and oral potentially malignant disorders: a systematic review. *Oral. Dis.* 2011;17 Suppl 1:58-72.

[101] Fonseca-Silva T, Farias LC, Cardoso CM, et al., Analysis of p16(CDKN2A) methylation and HPV-16 infection in oral mucosal dysplasia. *Pathobiology* 2012;79:94-100.

[102] Jayaprakash V, Reid M, Hatton E, et al., Human papillomavirus types 16 and 18 in epithelial dysplasia of oral cavity and oropharynx: a meta-analysis, 1985-2010. *Oral. Oncol.* 2011;47:1048-1054.

[103] Cardesa A, Nadal A. Carcinoma of the head and neck in the HPV era. *Acta Dermatovenerol. Alp. Panonica Adriat.* 2011;20:161-173.

[104] Fornatora M, Jones AC, Kerpel S, Freedman P. Human papillomavirus-associated oral epithelial dysplasia (koilocytic dysplasia): an entity of unknown biologic potential. *Oral. Surg. Oral. Med. Oral. Pathol. Oral. Radiol. Endod.* 1996;82:47-56.

[105] El-Mofty SK. HPV-related squamous cell carcinoma variants in the head and neck. *Head Neck Pathol.* 2012;6 Suppl 1:S55-62.

[106] Zheng ZM, Wang X. Regulation of cellular miRNA expression by human papillomaviruses. *Biochim. Biophys. Acta* 2011;1809:668-677.

[107] Li B, Hu Y, Ye F, Li Y, Lv W, Xie X. Reduced miR-34a expression in normal cervical tissues and cervical lesions with high-risk human papillomavirus infection. *Int. J. Gynecol. Cancer* 2010;20:597-604.

[108] Lajer CB, Garnaes E, Friis-Hansen L, et al., The role of miRNAs in human papilloma virus (HPV)-associated cancers: bridging between HPV-related head and neck cancer and cervical cancer. *Br. J. Cancer* 2012;106:1526-1534.

[109] Malumbres M. miRNAs and cancer: An epigenetics view. *Mol. Aspects Med.* 2012;34:863-874.

[110] Lee RC, Feinbaum RL, Ambros V. The C-elegans heterochronic gene lin-4 encodes small RNAs with antisense complementarity to lin-14. *Cell* 1993;75:843-854.

[111] McCullough MJ, Prasad G, Zhao S, Farah CS. The changing aetiology of oral cancer and the role of novel biomarkers to aid in early diagnosis. In: Ogbureke KUE, ed. Oral cancer. InTech, 2012:129-148. Available from: 'http://www.intechopen.com/books /oral-cancer/the-changing-aetiology-of-oral-cancer-and-the-role-of-novel-biomarkers-to-aid-in-early-diagnosis'.

[112] Gunawardena I, Fitzgerald J, Morley A, Hussey DJ, Woods CM, Carney AS. Micro-ribonucleic acids in head and neck cancer: an introduction. *J. Laryngol. Otol.* 2013;1-6.

[113] John K, Wu J, Lee BW, Farah CS. MicroRNAs in Head and Neck Cancer. *Int. J. Dent.* 2013;2013:650218.

[114] Nagadia R, Pandit P, Coman WB, Cooper-White J, Punyadeera C. miRNAs in head and neck cancer revisited. *Cell Oncol.* 2013;36:1-7.

[115] Wu BH, Xiong XP, Jia J, Zhang WF. MicroRNAs: new actors in the oral cancer scene. *Oral. Oncol.* 2011;47:314-319.

[116] Iorio MV, Croce CM. MicroRNA dysregulation in cancer: diagnostics, monitoring and therapeutics. A comprehensive review. *EMBO Mol. Med.* 2012;4:143-159.

[117] Gao G, Gay HA, Chernock RD, et al., A microRNA expression signature for the prognosis of oropharyngeal squamous cell carcinoma. *Cancer* 2013;119:72-80.

[118] Wald AI, Hoskins EE, Wells SI, Ferris RL, Khan SA. Alteration of microRNA profiles in squamous cell carcinoma of the head and neck cell lines by human papillomavirus. *Head Neck* 2011;33:504-512.

[119] Hui AB, Lin A, Xu W, et al., Potentially prognostic micro-RNAs in HPV-associated oropharyngeal carcinoma. *Clin. Cancer Res.* 2013;19:2154-2162.

[120] Lajer CB, Nielsen FC, Friis-Hansen L, et al., Different miRNA signatures of oral and pharyngeal squamous cell carcinomas: a prospective translational study. *Br. J. Cancer* 2011;104:830-840.

[121] Esquela-Kerscher A, Trang P, Wiggins JF, et al., The let-7 microRNA reduces tumor growth in mouse models of lung cancer. *Cell Cycle* 2008;7:759-764.

[122] Baek D, Villen J, Shin C, Camargo FD, Gygi SP, Bartel DP. The impact of microRNAs on protein output. *Nature* 2008;455:64-71.

[123] Selbach M, Schwanhaeusser B, Thierfelder N, Fang Z, Khanin R, Rajewsky N. Widespread changes in protein synthesis induced by microRNAs. *Nature* 2008;455:58-63.

[124] Gallagher IJ, Scheele C, Keller P, et al., Integration of microRNA changes in vivo identifies novel molecular features of muscle insulin resistance in type 2 diabetes. *Genome Med.* 2010;2:9.

[125] Roh J-L, Wang XV, Manola J, Sidransky D, Forastiere AA, Koch WM. Clinical correlates of promoter hypermethylation of four target genes in head and neck cancer: A cooperative group correlative study. *Clin. Cancer Res.* 2013;19:2528-2540.

[126] Kostareli E, Holzinger D, Hess J. New concepts for translational head and neck oncology: Lessons from HPV-related oropharyngeal squamous cell carcinomas. *Front Oncol.* 2012;2:1-10.

[127] Sartor MA, Dolinoy DC, Jones TR, et al., Genome-wide methylation and expression differences in HPV(+) and HPV(-) squamous cell carcinoma cell lines are consistent with divergent mechanisms of carcinogenesis. *Epigenetics* 2011;6:777-787.

[128] Richards KL, Zhang B, Baggerly KA, et al., Genome-wide hypomethylation in head and neck cancer is more pronounced in HPV-negative tumors and is associated with genomic instability. *PLoS One* 2009;4:1-7.

[129] Biron VL, Mohamed A, Hendzel MJ, Alan Underhill D, Seikaly H. Epigenetic differences between human papillomavirus-positive and -negative oropharyngeal squamous cell carcinomas. *J. Otolaryngol. Head Neck Surg.* 2012;41 Suppl 1:S65-70.

[130] O'Rorke MA, Ellison MV, Murray LJ, Moran M, James J, Anderson LA. Human papillomavirus related head and neck cancer survival: A systematic review and meta-analysis. *Oral. Oncol.* 2012;48:1191-1201.

[131] Worden FP, Kumar B, Lee JS, et al., Chemoselection as a strategy for organ preservation in advanced oropharynx cancer: Response and survival positively associated with HPV16 copy number. *J. Clin. Oncol.* 2008;26:3138-3146.

[132] Polanska H, Raudenska M, Gumulec J, et al., Clinical significance of head and neck squamous cell cancer biomarkers. *Oral. Oncology* 2014;50:168-177.

[133] Chen SF, Yu FS, Chang YC, Fu E, Nieh S, Lin YS. Role of human papillomavirus infection in carcinogenesis of oral squamous cell carcinoma with evidences of prognostic association. *J .Oral. Pathol. Med.* 2012;41:9-15.

[134] Balaram P, Nalinakumari KR, Abraham E, et al., Human papillomaviruses in 91 oral cancers from Indian betel quid chewers - High prevalence and multiplicity of infections. *Int. J. Cancer* 1995;61:450-454.
[135] Caussy D, Goedert JJ, Palefsky J, et al., Interaction of Human Immunodeficiency and Papilloma Viruses - Association with Anal Epithelial Abnormality in Homosexual Men. *Int. J. Cancer* 1990;46:214-219.
[136] Loyo M, Li RJ, Bettegowda C, et al., Lessons learned from next-generation sequencing in head and neck cancer. *Head Neck* 2012;35:454-463.
[137] Nygard M, Aagnes B, Bray F, Moller B, Mork J. Population-based evidence of increased survival in human papillomavirus-related head and neck cancer. *Eur. J. Cancer* 2012;48:1341-1346.
[138] Duray A, Descamps G, Decaestecker C, et al., Human papillomavirus DNA strongly correlates with a poorer prognosis in oral cavity carcinoma. *Laryngoscope* 2012;122:1558-1565.
[139] Dahlgren L, Mellin H, Wangsa D, et al., Comparative genomic hybridization analysis of tonsillar cancer reveals a different pattern of genomic imbalances in human papillomavirus-positive and -negative tumors. *Int. J. Cancer* 2003;107:244-249.
[140] Jung AC, Briolat J, Millon R, et al., Biological and clinical relevance of transcriptionally active human papillomavirus (HPV) infection in oropharynx squamous cell carcinoma. *Int. J. Cancer* 2010;126:1882-1894.
[141] Klussmann JP, Mooren JJ, Lehnen M, et al., Genetic signatures of HPV-related and unrelated oropharyngeal carcinoma and their prognostic implications. *Clin. Cancer Res.* 2009;15:1779-1786.
[142] Smeets SJ, Braakhuis BJ, Abbas S, et al., Genome-wide DNA copy number alterations in head and neck squamous cell carcinomas with or without oncogene-expressing human papillomavirus. *Oncogene* 2006;25:2558-2564.
[143] Wilting SM, Smeets SJ, Snijders PJ, et al., Genomic profiling identifies common HPV-associated chromosomal alterations in squamous cell carcinomas of cervix and head and neck. *BMC Med. Genomics* 2009;2:1-11.
[144] Gillison ML, Castellsague X, Chaturvedi A, et al., Eurogin 2012 roadmap: Comparative epidemiology of HPV infection and associated cancers of the head and neck and cervix. *Int. J. Cancer* 2013;134:497-507.
[145] Pignon JP, le Maitre A, Maillard E, Bourhis J. Meta-analysis of chemotherapy in head and neck cancer (MACH-NC): an update on 93 randomised trials and 17,346 patients. *Radiother Oncol.* 2009;92:4-14.
[146] Bonner JA, Harari PM, Giralt J, et al., Radiotherapy plus cetuximab for squamous-cell carcinoma of the head and neck. *N. Engl. J. Med.* 2006;354:567-578.
[147] Vermorken JB, Mesia R, Rivera F, et al., Platinum-based chemotherapy plus cetuximab in head and neck cancer. *N. Engl. J. Med.* 2008;359:1116-1127.
[148] Tang AL, Owen JH, Hauff SJ, et al., Head and neck cancer stem cells: The effect of HPV--an in vitro and mouse Study. *Otolaryngol. Head Neck Surg.* 2013;149 252-260.
[149] Vermeer DW, Spanos WC, Vermeer PD, Bruns AM, Lee KM, Lee JH. Radiation-induced loss of cell surface CD47 enhances immune-mediated clearance of human papillomavirus-positive cancer. *Int. J. Cancer* 2013;133:120-129.

In: Head and Neck Cancer
Editor: Madison R. Hall

ISBN: 978-1-63482-113-1

Chapter 6

Epstein-Barr Virus Status and LMP1 Oncogene Polymorphism in Patients with Nasopharyngeal Carcinoma and Other Tumors of the Oral Cavity in a Non-Endemic Region

N. Senyuta, E. Goncharova, V. Kondratova, L. Scherback, K. Smirnova, V. Vayradyan, M. Lomaya, D. Maksimovich, A. Lichtenstein and V. Gurtsevitch
FSBI N.N. Blokhin Cancer Research Center, RAMS, Moscow, Russia

Abstract

The role of the Epstein-Barr virus (EBV), a ubiquitous lymphotropic human herpesvirus type 4, in the development of different tumours is not fully understood. In particular, it is unclear whether a specific strain or any strain of EBV circulating in the population is involved in carcinogenesis.

Elucidation of this problem for non-endemic regions, such as Russia, where EBV-associated tumours arise sporadically, is especially important. The present study aimed to study the status of EBV infection as well as the genetic structure of *LMP1* (a key oncogene of the virus) in patients with nasopharyngeal carcinoma (NPC) and in patients with other tumours of the oral cavity (OTOC). To this end, a comparative analysis of virus-specific antibody levels and the number of EBV DNA copies in the plasma of 22 NPC patients, 17 patients with OTOC and 19 blood donors (BDs) were tested. Special attention was paid to the investigation of polymorphisms of LMP1 in samples derived from tumour biopsies, blood lymphocytes and/or oropharyngeal lavages collected from the tested groups. The data reveal the presence of significantly higher anti-EBV antibody titres in the plasma of NPC compared to OTOC patients, but the number of DNA copies of the virus in the compared patient groups did not differ significantly. The analysis of the C-terminal region of the LMP1 sequences revealed that they closely matched LMP1 variants previously described by Edwards et al. (1999).

However, some characteristic features were also detected. In particular, the G212S substitution was not observed at all in the investigated LMP1 isolates. Overall, LMP1 variants from tumour samples of NPC and OTOC patients did not differ significantly either in the frequency of "highly oncogenic" LMP1 samples with 10 aa and/or 23 aa deletions (LMP1^{China1} and/or LMP1^{Med+}), nor in the number of 11 aa repeats and the frequency of 5 aa motif insertions. No statistically significant differences were detected in the frequency of amino acid substitutions between LMP1 samples obtained from tumour biopsies and oropharyngeal lavages of both patient groups. Structurally similar LMP1 variants observed in both groups of patients are likely to reflect the polymorphism of EBV strains circulating in the general population. These data may indicate that, in both NPC and OTOC patients, EBV strains with similar LMP1 variants are found to persist. This observation allows us to suggest that, at least in non-endemic areas, EBV strains with any LMP1variants can induce NPC development, but the oncogenic potential of the virus in an infected individual may be realised only in the presence of additional exposure to harmful factors in the internal and external environment, such as chemical carcinogens, congenital or acquired immunodeficiency, a genetic predisposition to NPC development, and possibly dietary and other factors. To confirm the above assumption, a comprehensive and long-term study in several population groups with high and low levels of EBV-associated pathologies should be carried out.

Keywords: Epstein-Barr virus (EBV), nasopharyngeal carcinoma (NPC), other tumours of the oral cavity (OTOC), anti-EBV antibody titers EBV DNA copies in blood plasma, phylogenetic analysis, LMP1 polymorphism, Russian patients

Introduction

Epstein-Barr virus (EBV), a member of the herpesvirus family, is an infectious agent that infects more than 90% of the adult population of the world. Despite the ubiquitous nature of the virus' distribution, it does not cause the majority of virus carriers any clinical symptoms, although in some cases, it may be the etiologic agent for a wide variety of malignant neoplasms of lymphoid and epithelial origin, including Burkitt's lymphoma (BL), Hodgkin's lymphoma (HL), nasopharyngeal carcinoma (NPC), certain cases of stomach cancer (SC) and many others [1]. Some EBV-associated malignancies, like NPC, are characterised by limited geographical and racial distribution [2, 3]. Being a rare disease in most countries of the world, NPC is found with an average frequency in the Arab countries of North Africa and Alaska and is considered to be endemic in the southern provinces in China and some other countries of Southeast Asia [4]. The reasons for the high incidence of EBV-associated NPC cases in certain geographic regions have not yet been elucidated. At the same time, we cannot exclude the impact of a number of factors on this process, namely the circulation in endemic regions of highly pathogenic EBV strains, a genetic predisposition of the population in these territories to NPC development and exposure to a number of harmful factors in the internal and external environment. The reasons for the appearance of NPC in non-endemic regions are an even greater mystery. In particular, it is not clear what role EBV plays in the pathogenesis of this disease.

As shown by numerous studies, the unique ability of EBV to transform infected cells is dependent on the function of a key viral protein, latent membrane protein 1 (LMP1) [5]. It is also known that this process is carried out through the interaction of LMP1 with a nuclear viral protein that also possesses transforming ability, EBNA2 [6]. Structurally, LMP1 is an integral membrane phosphoprotein with a molecular mass of 63 kDa, which consists of a 23-membered cytoplasmic N-terminal domain (NTD), six hydrophobic transmembrane domains (TMD) (163 amino acid residues), and a long cytoplasmic C-terminal domain (CTD) (200 amino acid residues) [7]. The LMP1 CTD includes three C-terminal transactivating regions (CTAR). Both the proximal CTAR1 (amino acid residues 194–232) and distal CTAR2 (amino acid residues 351–386) regions are responsible for the activation of a number of cellular signal cascades, which determines the significance of these LMP1 regions in terms of transforming potential [8, 9]. The CTAR3 region (amino acid residues 275–330), located between CTAR1 and CTAR2, presumably recruits JAK3, which results in STAT3 activation. This LMP1 region (as opposed to CTAR1 and CTAR2) is involved in the transforming growth of B lymphocytes [7, 10, 11]. It has been demonstrated that LMP1 expression results in the transformation of rodent fibroblasts and human B lymphocytes in vitro, as well as in the development of lymphomas in transgenic mice [12].

Global interest in LMP1 was largely stimulated by a number of reports about the detection of protein variants that determine an aggressive, geographically limited EBV phenotype. In particular, the cloning and sequencing of LMP1 samples from NPC patients in China showed in one sample a few mutations that are absent in the wild (prototype) LMP1 strain of EBV, B95.8 [13]. This naturally occurring variant of LMP1, called Cao (404 aa residues), has a deletion of 10 aa adjacent to the CTAR2 region and a 26 amino acid substitution in all domains of LMP1. Later, highly transforming LMP1 variants (like Chinese Cao) were isolated from NPC patients in Taiwan (C15) and the Mediterranean region (T510) [14-16].

The study of the polymorphisms of the LMP1 gene and possible associations with EBV-associated diseases has yielded important information about the existence of different isoforms of this gene, which allows them to be classified into groups [17-20]. Sandvej et al. [18] distributed all samples of gene isolates they studied into four main groups called A, B, C, and D. The members of group A carry six single substitutions in the gene and a single substitution in the promoter and, thus, are identical to the prototype LMP1 variant B95-8 (B95-8/A). The number of mutations is larger and more diverse in the members of other groups. It is important to note that even variants of group A, as well as members of other groups, contain several Cao-specific amino acid substitutions, such as I85L, F106Y, G212S, and S366T. In addition, most isolates that belong to these groups have additional random mutations. Based on the LMP1 samples amplified from patients with EBV-associated pathology and healthy individuals from different geographic regions, Edwards et al. [17] suggested their own classification of LMP1 variants using the frequency of their geographical detection (Alaskan, China 1 (Ch1), China 2 (Ch2), China 3 (Ch3), Mediterranean + (Med+), Mediterranean – (Med–) and North Carolina (NC)). Subsequent studies demonstrated that the frequency of these variants also varies considerably among the different pathologies associated with EBV.

Taking into account that the role of EBV in the origin of NPC remains poorly studied, the elucidation of this problem for non-endemic regions, such as Russia, where EBV-associated tumours arise sporadically, is especially important. The present study aimed to find genetic differences between EBV strains circulating in patients with EBV-associated forms of NPC, on the one hand, and viral strains persisting in patients with non- EBV-associated tumours localised in the oral cavity, on the other hand. A comparison of the genetic structure of the LMP1 oncogene in biological specimens from both patients groups under investigation allowed us to conclude whether common strains persisting in the local population or specific EBV strains are associated with NPC in a non-endemic region such as Russia.

Materials and Methods

Patient Characteristics and Clinical Samples

The investigated samples were tumour biopsies, blood and/or oropharyngeal lavages collected from 22 patients with nasopharyngeal carcinoma (NPC) and 17 patients with other (non- nasopharyngeal carcinoma) tumours of the oral cavity (OTOC), as well as blood samples obtained from 19 blood donors (BDs). The other tumours of the oral cavity included cancers of the mucous membrane of the tongue (three cases), floor of the mouth (two cases), cheek (one case), retro molar area (three cases), lower jaw (four cases) and palate (five cases).

The diagnosis of undifferentiated NPC was confirmed histologically and cytologically based on WHO criteria. The overwhelming majority of patients were in advanced stages of the disease (III and IV) and in the process of chemotherapy or chemo-radiotherapy. The average age of both groups of patients was identical and equal to 50.4 years. The average age in the group of BDs was 48.7 years. The Ethical Committee at the Russian N.N. Blokhin Cancer Research Centre approved the present study, which included randomly selected patients with nasopharyngeal carcinomas and other non-nasopharyngeal carcinoma tumours with their informed consent.

DNA Extraction and Sequence Analysis of PCR Products

DNA from the biological specimens collected (tumour biopsies, blood cells and throat lavage) was extracted by phenol-chloroform deproteinisation. The presence of human DNA in all specimens was evaluated by means of real-time PCR with primers to the reference *GAPDH* gene: 5′-AGT CCA GTG AGC TTC CCG TTC AGC-3′; 5′-TGG TAT CGT GGA AGG ACT CAT GAC-3′ and SYBR Green 1 dye (1:75,000 dilutions). Amplification was carried out using the following cycling schedule: denaturation at 94°C for 2 min, then 50 cycles of 94°C for 20 s, 64°C for 20 s, and 72°C for 10 s. The reactions were run in 96-well plates using an iQ5 Real-Time PCR detection system (Bio-Rad Labs, Hercules, CA). Each DNA sample was then screened for the presence of *LMP1* using “nested” PCR with primers designed to amplify the C-terminal fragment (aa 212-387):

external – Eco3′: 5′- TCCAGGAGAATTCCCCATCTCGAGAGTG-3′ and 8785: 5′-CGACCCCAATCTGGATGTATTATTATGG-3′;

internal – Bam3′: 5′-GTTTTCGTGGATCCTTATACAGTA-3′ and
8702: 5′-GCTACCGATTCTGGCCATGAATCTGAC-3′, as described [21]. Each PCR product was purified on a QIAGEN mini-column (QIAGEN in Russian Fed., Moscow)

according to the instructions of the manufacturer. As a positive control, 100 ng of DNA isolated from the B95-8 cell line was used. Each sample was analysed in duplicate. Negative water blanks were included in every analysis. LMP1 amplicons were sequenced in both directions. DNA sequencing was done by means of a panel of ABI PRISM® BigDye™ Terminator reagents, v. 3.1, with subsequent analysis of reaction products on an automatic DNA sequencer ABI PRISM 3100-Avant. Data processing was done using Chromas 230 and Vector NTI software.

Quantitative Determination of the Number of EBV DNA Copies

The amount of viral DNA copies in 1 mL of plasma was determined by real-time PCR. DNA from Namalwa diploid cells (that contain two integrated viral genomes) was used for the construction of calibration curves; it was based on the ratio of 3.3 pg genomic DNA per 1 copy of viral DNA [22]. For real-time PCR, the primers to the 76 bp fragment in the BamHIW region of viral DNA (GenBank ID: V01555) were used, including the sense primer W44F (5'_CCCAACACTCCACCACACC), antisense primer W-119R (5'-TCTTAGGAG CTGTCCGAGGG), and fluorescent probe W-67T (5'-FAM-CACACACTACACACACCC ACCCGTCTC-RTQ1) [23]. The possibility of using blood plasma DNA as a matrix in PCR was estimated by taking the unique *K-RAS* gene as a control as described previously [24]. The reaction was conducted in 96-well plates on a CFX96 device (Bio-Rad Laboratories, United States) in 50 μL of reaction mixture (Syntol, Russia) containing 0.3 μM of each primer, 25 nM fluorescent probe, 4 mM $MgCl_2$, 200 mM of each dNTP, 1 unit of Taq polymerase and 10 μL of DNA solution in a 10 mM Tris HCl buffer, pH 8.0, with 1 mM EDTA (corresponding to 50 μL of plasma).

Two negative controls (samples that did not contain DNA) were included in each analysis. PCR conditions were as follows: denaturation at 95°C (5 min), the 40 cycles at 95°C for 15 s and 56.5°C for 30 s. Data from real-time PCR were analysed using the CFX Manager program (Bio-Rad).

Determination of the Serological Response to EBV Antigens

The titres of IgG antibodies to the viral capsid (VCA), early (RA) and nuclear 1 (EBNA1) antigens and IgA antibodies to the same EBV antigens were measured in the plasma of NPC and OTOC patients, as well as in BDs by an indirect immunofluorescence assay; the conditions and the analysis of the results from this assay have been described previously [25]. Antibody titres are expressed as their geometric mean (GMT) value.

Phylogenetic Analysis

The nucleotide sequences of LMP1 samples obtained from the analysed specimens were translated into amino acid (aa) sequences corresponding to codons 212–387 of the B95.8 prototype strain (NCBI, X01995) with the vector NTI software package (Invitrogen, Carlsbad, CA). Distance matrices were calculated using the Kimura-2 parameter model and a phylogenetic tree was constructed from these distance matrices using the neighbour-joining (NJ) program. Phylogenetic analysis was conducted using MEGA version 2.1.

Statistical Analysis

Fisher's exact test was used to compare the prevalence of LMP1 isolates between different specimens from NPC and OTOC patients and BDs. P-values less than 0.05 were considered to indicate significant differences. The equivalence of the mean percentages of aa substitutions in LMP1 isolates obtained from the two groups of patients (NPC and OTOC) was determined by t-tests. The statistical package STATA was used (StataCorp. 1999. Stata Statistical Software: Release 6.0. College Station, Texas: Stata Corporation).

Results and Discussion

EBV-Specific Antibodies in Blood Plasma

One of the indications of a pronounced association between NPC and EBV is the detection of a strong serological response to viral antigens in NPC patients [1, 25].

It should be noted that high titres of antibodies to EBV are frequently detected many years before the disease occurs, while in many cases, an increase or decrease in these titres reflects the dynamics of the tumour process (recurrence or remission) [4]. In our study, titres of IgG antibodies to VCA and RA viral antigens in the blood plasma of NPC patients were typically high, much higher than the corresponding values of antibody titres in OTOC patients (Table 1).

The titres of IgA antibodies to the same EBV antigens in patients with NPC also exceeded those in OTOC patients by several times. In blood donors, antibody titres were low, even lower than the corresponding titres in OTOC patients. Thus, despite the fact that NPC is not endemic in Russia, this tumour is closely associated with EBV in this country, while the association with the virus was not serologically detected for patients with OTOC.

Quantitative Analysis of Circulating Cell-Free EBV DNA in Blood Plasma

The higher antibody titres to EBV antigens detected in NPC patients apparently suggest higher concentrations of viral DNA copies circulating in the plasma of these patients. To verify the assumed correlations, quantitative analysis of circulating cell-free EBV DNA was carried out in the plasma of the two patient groups and BD. Using real-time quantitative PCR, the median plasma EBV DNA concentration in 23 NPC patients was determined to be 9100 copies/ml, whereas that in 26 healthy controls was 980 copies/ml, $P < 0.05$ (Figure 1).

Unexpectedly, the concentration of EBV DNA in plasma of 13 OTOC patients (in spite of the low serological response to the virus) was rather similar to that in the plasma of NPC patients (8300 copies/ml vs. 9100 copies/ml, $P > 0.05$).

Table 1. Serological response to Epstein-Barr virus (EBV) antigens in NPC and OTOC patients and BDs

mmunoglobulin's classes	IgG			IgA		
EBV antigens	VCA	EA	EBNA1	VCA	EA	EBNA1
Antibody response to EBV antigens in NPC patients						
Number of patients examined	21	21	21	21	19	21
Percentage of seropositive patients	100	100	100	100	52.6	95.2
Geometric mean value of antibody titers	1085.3	271.3	92.0	131.4	99,6	12,6
Antibody response to EBV antigens in OTOC patients						
Number of patients examined	20	20	18	20	20	18
Percentage of seropositive patients	90,0	30,0	94.4	10.0	0	11.1
Geometric mean value of antibody titers	86,4	25,2	8.7	28,3	0	5,7
Antibody response to EBV antigens in blood donors						
Number of tested blood donors	25	25	nt	25	25	nt
Percentage of seropositive patients	96,0	8,0	nt	0	0	nt
Geometric mean value of antibody titers	22,1	10,0	nt	0	0	nt

Antibody titers to the capsid (VCA), early (EA) and nuclear (EBNA) EBV antigens were determined using a ten-fold (for detection anti VCA and EA antibodies) and two-fold (for detection anti-EBNA antibody) dilutions of the plasma.

nt - Plasma samples for the presence of EBV-specific antibodies in these groups was not tested.

NPC - nasopharyngeal carcinoma; OTOC - other tumours of the oral cavity; BDs – blood donors.

These data differ from those described by Lo and others [23, 26, 27] who observed a significantly higher EBV load in NPC patients compared to OTOC patients. A possible explanation of our findings could be massive infiltration of non-EBV-associated tumours of the oral cavity with EBV-infected B lymphocytes, most of which were subjected to lytic EBV infection. As shown, the enhanced proliferation of EBV-infected B lymphocytes is due tumour production of proinflammatory cytokines such as interleukin-6 and granulocyte-macrophage colony-stimulating factor [28, 29]. The higher EBV DNA concentrations in the blood plasma of our healthy individuals, as compared to levels shown in other studies, may also be associated with some benign inflammatory condition or infection at the time of blood collection [30]. We can also assume that the increased concentration of EBV DNA in the plasma of OTOC patients and healthy individuals involved in this study is due to their genetic predisposition to increased replicative EBV activity. A relatively small number of observations could also affect the results of this study.

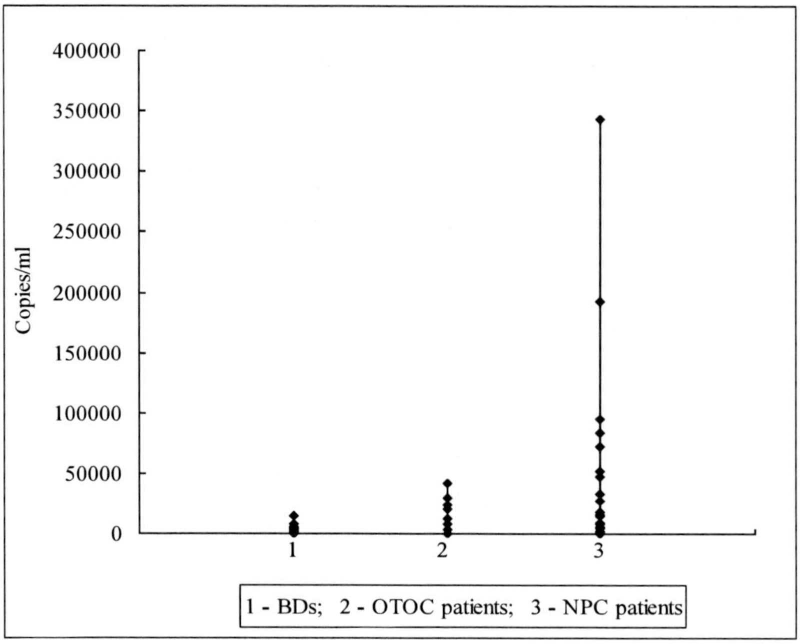

BDs – blood donors; OTOC - patients with other tumours of the oral cavity;
NPC - patients with nasopharyngeal carcinoma.

Figure 1. Detection of plasma cell-free EBV DNA copies in NPC and OTOC patients and BDs.

The categories: NPC and OTOC patients (26 subjects and 13 subjects, respectively) as well as BDs (26 control subjects) tested for EBV DNA copies in blood plasma samples are plotted on the X axis. Results are indicated by ♦. The Y axis denotes the concentration of cell-free EBV DNA (copies of EBV DNA/ml of plasma) detected in each subjects by the BamHIW region real-time quantitative PCR.

Additional studies are required to assess the diagnostic and prognostic values of EBV DNA plasma levels as a tumour marker for patients with different oral cavity tumours in non-endemic regions.

Pattern of LMP1 Variants in Biological Specimens of NPC and OTOC Patients

An analysis of the nucleotide and predicted amino acid (aa) sequences in LMP1 amplicons revealed some variability (Table 2), but in general they matched the LMP1 variants that have been described previously: B95.8/A, Cao/China1, Mediterranean plus and minus (Med+, Med–), and North Carolina (NC) [18–20]. Four LMP1 samples that did not match any of the variants in the above-mentioned classifications were designated as "OC" (outside of classification). All of them were amplified from samples taken from NPC patients (two from tumour tissue, one from blood, and one from an oropharyngeal lavage).

It is also evident from the Table 2 that the low-divergent $LMP1^{B95.8/A}$ variant, which is characterised by a small number (3-4) of aa substitutions (in comparison with the prototype $LMP1^{B95.8}$ variant) and low transforming activity was predominant in blood donor samples, accounting for 78.9% (15/19) of all variant; this was less frequently observed in samples from NPC (27.3%, 6/22) and OTOC (14.3%, 2/14) patients. The differences between the values obtained in blood donor samples and those for both types of tumour samples approached statistical significance (P=0.105 and P=0.0526, respectively).

Importantly, in 15 blood samples from NPC patients, the $LMP1^{China1}$ variant (the analogue of the Chinese LMP1Cao strain characterised by high transforming activity) was not detected in any case, while in blood samples from OTOC patients, it was detected in 66.7% (8/12) of cases. The sum of the $LMP1^{China1}$ + $LMP1^{Med+}$ variants (both variants are highly divergent ones and contain a deletion of 10 aa) that originated from blood samples from NPC patients was also significantly lower than that from blood samples from OTOC patients ((13.3% (2/15) vs. 75.0% (9/12), respectively), and the difference between the values obtained approached statistical significance (P = 0.072)).

As shown in Table 2, the frequency of the detection of the "highly tumorigenic" $LMP1^{China1}$ variant [Blake et al., 2001; Miller et al., 1998], the analogue of the Chinese $LMP1^{Cao}$ strain [Edwards et al., 1999; Miller et al., 1994], was higher in biopsies of other tumours of the oral cavity (35.7%, 5/14) in comparison with NPC samples (9.1%, 2/22).

Table 2. Spectrum of LMP1 variants derived from tumour biopsies, blood samples and oropharyngeal lavages of NPC and OTOC patients and peripheral blood lymphocytes of BDs

Tested specimens	Tested groups	LMP1 variants[1]					
		B95.8/A (%)	China1 (%)	Med+ (%)	Med- (%)	NC (%)	OC[2] (%)
Tumour biopsies	NPC n=22	6 (27.3)	2 (9.1)	8 (36.4)	3 (3.6)	1 (4.5)	2 (9.1)
	OTOC n=14	2 (14.3)	5 (35.7)	3 (21.4)	2 (14.3)	2 (14.3)	0 (0.0)
Blood samples	NPC n=15	3 (20.0)	0 (0.0)	2 (13.3)	7 (46.7)	2 (13.3)	1 (6.7)
	OTOC n=12	1 (8,3)	8 (66.7)	1 (8.3)	1 (8.3)	1 (8.3)	0 (0.0)
	Blood donors n=19	15 (78.9)	1 (5.3)	0 (0.0)	1 (5.3)	2 (10.5)	0 (0.0)
Oropharyngeal lavages	NPC n=19	6 (31.6)	0 (0.0)	6 (31.6)	4 (21.0)	2 (15.8)	1 (5.3)
	OTOC n=9	2 (22.2)	3 (33.3)	1 (11.1)	2 (22.2)	1 (11.1)	0 (0.0)

[1]LMP1 - samples amplified from NPC and OTOC patients and PBL of BDs were evaluated as variants according to classification suggested by Sandvej et al. 1997 and Edwards et al., 1999.

[2]OC (outside of classification) – LMP1 samples characterized by a specific set of mutations that differed from all previously described LMP1 variants.

NPC - patients with nasopharyngeal carcinoma; OTOC - patients with other tumours of the oral cavity; BDs – blood donors.

The total sum of all LMP1 variants containing the 10 aa deletion (i.e. China1 and Med+) derived from NPC specimens (45.5%, 10/22) was lower than from other tumours of the oral cavity (57.1%, 8/14); however, the difference between these values was not statistically significant.

The difference between the joint frequencies of $LMP1^{Med-}$ and $LMP1^{NC}$ variants (regarded as "poorly tumorigenic") derived from tumour samples from NPC and OTOC patients was also not statistically significant (18.2% (4/22) and 28.6% (4/14), respectively), despite the fact that the frequency of the $LMP1^{NC}$ variant was higher in OTOC patients than that in NPC patients (14.3% (2/14) vs. 4.5% (1/22), respectively).

The total sum of the "poorly tumorigenic" $LMP1^{Med-}$ and $LMP1^{NC}$ variants derived from the blood samples of NPC patients was higher than that derived from the blood samples of OTOC patients (60.0% (9/15) vs. 16.7% (2/12), respectively), although the difference was not statistically significant (P=0.16).

The distribution pattern of LMP1 variants originating from oropharyngeal lavages of NPC and OTOC patients resembled that observed from blood samples of the same patients: the frequency of deleted LMP1 variants (i.e. China1 and Med+) obtained from oropharyngeal lavages of patients with OTOC was slightly higher (44.4%, 4/9) than that originating from oropharyngeal lavages of NPC patients (31.6%, 6/19); the difference was statistically insignificant. The value of frequencies of $LMP1^{Med-}$ and $LMP1^{NC}$ variants derived from oropharyngeal lavages of NPC (21.0%, 4/19 and 15.8%, 2/19) and OTOC (11.1%, 1/9 and 22.2%, 2/9) patients did not differ significantly.

The data obtained suggest that the development of NPC in a non-endemic region (Russia) is not related to the spread of "highly tumorigenic" EBV strains carrying $LMP1^{China1}$ and/or $LMP1^{Med+}$ variants with the 10 aa deletion. These virus strains were predominantly present in specimens of patients with other tumours of the oral cavity and occasionally in peripheral lymphocytes of blood donors. This assumption is in line with the conclusion of other investigators who believe that the high incidence of NPC in Southern China is unlikely to be due to the high prevalence of EBV strains carrying the $LMP1^{Cao}$ variant in that community [Leung et al., 1997; Shu, Tu, 2000; Zhang et al., 2002].

Moreover, the current study demonstrates that EBV strains with any variant of the LMP1 gene are persistent in tumours, either associated or not associated with EBV (NPC and OTOC, respectively), and their spectrum did not differ between patient groups.

Deleted LMP1 Variants in NPC and OTOC Patients

The tumorigenic and transforming features of LMP1 are usually associated with the 10 aa/30 bp deletion [7, 31], which is sometimes located within the overlapping part of 23 aa/69 bp deletion. In connection with this, it was of interest to compare the frequency of the above deletions in LMP1 samples derived from NPC and OTOC patients. Sequence analysis of LMP1 isolates derived from 22 NPC biopsies found four LMP1 samples (18.2%) with the 10 aa/30 bp deletion (spanning codons 346-355), six LMP1 samples (27.3%) with the 23 aa/69 bp deletion (spanning codons 334-355, covering the 10 aa deletion); the other 12 LMP1 samples (54.5%) were undeleted (Table 3).

Table 3. The 10 and 23 aa deleted variants and key amino acid substitutions in LMP1 samples derived from tumor, blood and oropharyngeal lavage samples of NPC and OTOC patients and peripheral blood lymphocytes of BDs

Tested specimens	Tested groups	10 aa deletion (aa 346-355)	23 aa deletion (aa 334-356)	366 S→T/A	212 G→S
Tumour biopsies	NPC[a] (n=22)	4 (18.2%)	6 (27.3%)	S→T (59.0%), S→A (40.9%)	ND[1]
	OTOC (n=14)	7 (50.0%)	1 (7.1%)	S→T (100%), S→A (0.0%)	ND
Blood samples	NPC (n=15)	1 (6.7%)	1 (6.7%)	S→T (73.3%), S→A (26.7%)	ND
	OTOC (n=12	9 (75.0%)	0 (0.0%)	S→T (100%), S→A (0.0%)	ND
	BDs (n=19)	1 (5.3%)	0 (0.0%)	S→T (100%), S→A (0.0%)	ND
Oropharyn-geal lavages	NPC (n=19)	1 (5.3%)	5 (36.3%)	S→T (52.6%), S→A (47.4%)	ND
	OTOC (n=9)	4 (44.4%)	0 (0.0%)	S→T (100%), S→A (0.0%)	ND

LMP1 samples detected from tumour, blood and oropharyngeal lavage specimens of NPC and OTOC patients were grouped according to previously suggested classifications by Sandvej et al. 1997 and Edwards et al., 1999, and their percentage within each group tested is shown.

[1] ND–No amino acid substitution G→S at position 212 was detected.

NPC - patients with nasopharyngeal carcinoma; OTOC - patients with other tumours of the oral cavity; BDs – blood donors.

The results of the sequence analysis carried out for LMP1 isolates originating from 14 OTOC biopsies was different: LMP1 samples with the 10 aa/30 bp deletion were detected in seven cases (50.0%), while one case had the 23 aa/69 bp deletion (7.1%); the other six cases were undeleted (42.9%). However, the difference between the frequency of 10 aa and 23 aa deleted LMP1 samples obtained from tumour samples in the two patient groups was not statistically significant (45.5%, 10/22 vs. 57.1%, 8/14; P= 0.211).

In addition, it was found that LMP1 samples derived from tumour biopsies in both patient groups contained common aa substitutions clustered between codons 309 and 366: S309N, Q322E/N/D, E328Q/A, Q334/R, L338S/P, H352R/N and S366T/A. Interestingly, the LMP1 isolate with an S→T substitution at codon 366, common for NPC patients in endemic regions, was also common in our study (100%) in OTOC patients. However, for NPC patients, a rather high percentage of the S→A substitution was observed in tumour biopsies (40.9%, 9/22), blood samples (26.7%, 4/15) and oropharyngeal lavages (47.4%, 9/19). Another specific feature of Russian LMP1 isolates was a complete absence of the G→S substitution at codon 212 (Table 3), which has been described for different EBV-associated malignancies [32, 33].

Phylogenetic Analysis

To analyse the phylogenetic relationships between LMP1 isolates obtained from tumour samples of NPC and OTOC patients, 35 LMP1 nucleotide sequences (21 from NPC and 14 from OTOC) were determined and aligned. The prototype B95.8 and Cao LMP1 strain alignments were used for comparison. According to sequence variations, the LMP1 samples under investigation were classified into five variants and corresponding clusters were generated in the phylogenetic tree: B95.8/A, China 1, Med+, Med-, NC and OC (Figure 2). As shown by the phylogenetic tree, the LMP1^{Med+} variant was more common among nasopharyngeal carcinoma samples, while the LMP1^{China1} variant was more frequently detected among samples of patients with OTOC. In the phylogenetic tree, however, these two clusters of LMP1 samples were located quite distant one from another. The Med-, NC and B95.8/A clusters were relatively equally represented by LMP1 samples from the tumours of both patient groups. Two LMP1^{OC} samples, which did not relate to any classification in the phylogenetic tree, were located quite close to the B95.8/A cluster. In the phylogenetic tree, the confidence values for these samples were assessed by bootstrap analysis [34].

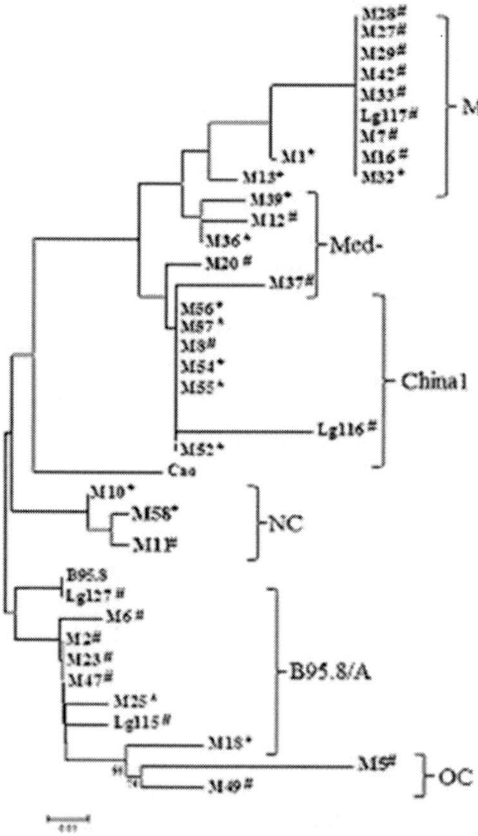

The phylogenetic tree was drawn from the C-terminal amino acid sequences of LMP1 samples obtained from tumor biopsies of NPC (n=22) and OTOC (n=17) patients by neighbor –joining method. These samples were grouped according to suggested classifications for LMP1 variants. The scale shown in the lower left reflect the evolutionary distance. #, LMP1 samples from NPC patients; *, LMP1 samples from patients with OTOC; OC - LMP1 samples outside of known classifications.

Figure 2. Phylogenetic analyses of the tumor-derived LMP1 variants from NPC and OTOC patients.

Repeat and Insertion Elements in LMP1

It has been shown that the C-terminal domain of different LMP1 isolates contains various numbers of 11 aa (PQDPDNTDDNG) repeats located between aa 253 and 306 [7, 32, 33].

The prototype LMP1B95.8 strain contains four such repeats and two 5 aa sequence insertions (PHDPL: 275–279): one is located between repeats 2 and 3, and the other after the last repeat (aa: 302–306). The 5 aa insertion represents the so-called JAK3-site of CTAR3 (aa: 275–330), which is presumably associated with activation of the JAK3/STAT signalling pathway [7, 32].

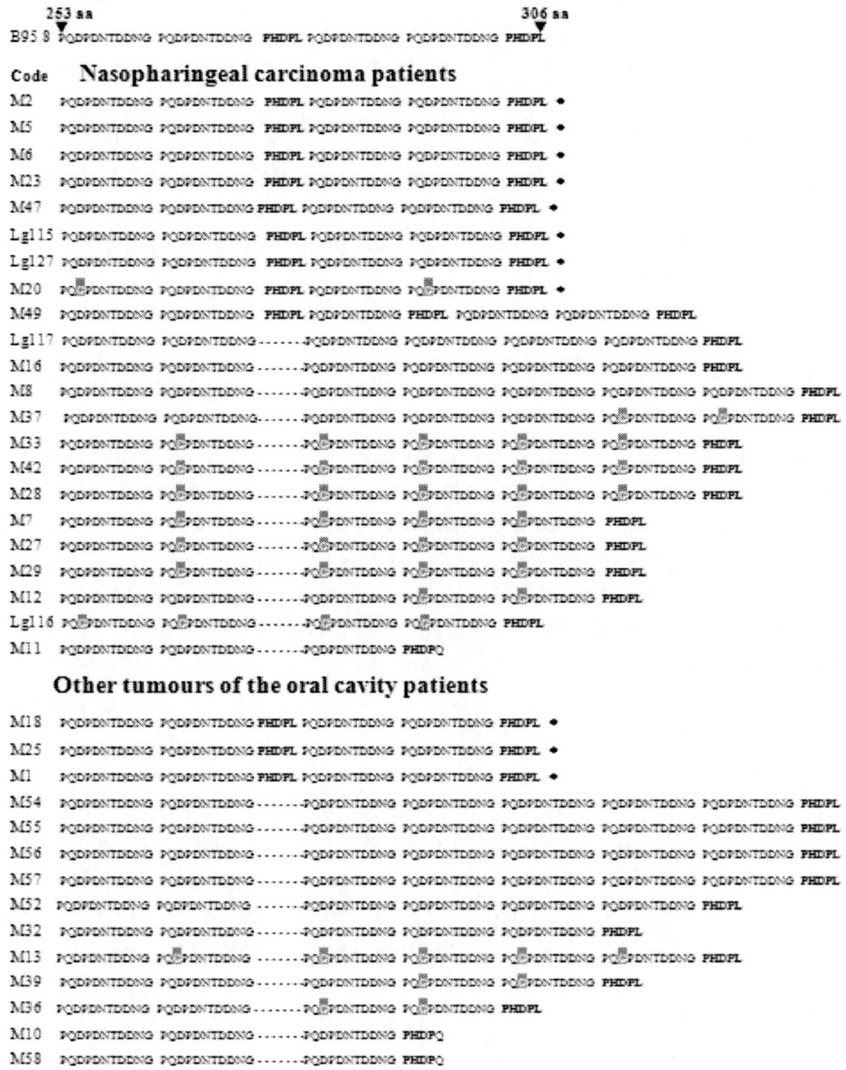

The pattern of 11 aa repeat elements (PQDPDNTDDNG) between aa 253 and 306 in the C -terminal domain of prototype B95.8 LMP1 is shown on the first line. The marks in the left column refer to individual isolates. PQDPDNTDDNG – 11 aa repeat element; PQ**G**PDNTDDNG – 11 aa repeat element with point mutation D→G; PHDPL, five amino acid sequence; *, LMP, sequence, which are identical to the prototype LMP1$^{B95.8}$ strain.

Figure 3. Variations in the 11 aa repeat elements and 5 aa sequence in the C-termini of LMP1 samples obtained from tumor specimens of NPC and OTOC patients.

To clarify the structural relationships between LMP1 samples obtained from tumour biopsies of nasopharyngeal carcinoma and other tumours of the oral cavity, their C-terminal domains were compared with respect to their combination of repeats and insertions (Figure 3).

The results indicate that, among the LMP1 samples originating from nasopharyngeal carcinoma and other tumours of the oral cavity, the percentages of B95-8-like sequences with the 5 aa insertion at position 275–279 did not differ significantly (40.9% (9/22), vs. 21.4% (3/14), P> 0.05, respectively).

All LMP1 samples, irrespective of their tumour origin, contained three to seven 11 aa repeats (PQDPDNTDDNG), making these samples similar to LMP1 samples from Africa and Japan [35]. However, unlike Japanese isolates, in LMP1 samples of Russian origin, the point mutation D→G was frequently found and more frequently in tumour samples from NPC patients than in tumour samples from OTOC patients (45.5% (10/22) and 21.4% (3/14), respectively), although the difference was not statistically significant. Analysing the data, it can be assumed that the formation of 11 aa repeats as well as 5 aa motif insertions may occur either by recombination events taking place during replication of the virus or due to some geographic specificity in the EBV structure, and probably do not play a crucial role in the biological functions of LMP1 [36, 37].

Range of LMP1 Variants in Different Specimens of the Same Patients

Several studies have shown that individuals can be infected with multiple EBV strains, apparently acquired at the time of primary infection [38-40]. A comparison of the range of LMP1 samples originated from tumour biopsies with those from blood and/or oropharyngeal lavages of the same nasopharyngeal carcinoma patients and patients with other tumours of the oral cavity revealed several patterns (Table 4). The number of cases with non-matching LMP1 samples (and, accordingly, LMP1 variants) obtained from tumours, on the one hand, and from blood and/or oropharyngeal lavage samples, on the other, was higher for NPC than for OTOC patients, but the difference between the compared values was not statistically significant (68.2% (15/22) vs. 23.1% (3/13); P= 0.206). The higher percentage of mismatched LMP1 variants detected for nasopharyngeal carcinoma specimens could be explained either by genetic predisposition of NPC patients to co-infection with several EBV strains leading to homologous recombination, or the enhanced replication of a primary acquired EBV strain in these individuals. Either of these events could lead to numerous mutations in the viral genome (and, accordingly, in the LMP1 gene) and, as a result, to the generation of EBV strain(s) with distinct LMP1 samples. On the other hand, the diversity of LMP1 samples may follow from mutations in EBV strains, which might result from immune selection phenomena that could be different in the two groups of patients [18, 41, 42] [Edwards et al., 2004, Deng et al., 2012, Lo et al., 2012].

The Search for Tumour-Specific LMP1 Variant(s)

To find tumour-specific LMP1 variant(s) in the tested NPC cases, LMP1 samples derived from tumour, blood and oropharyngeal lavages of nasopharyngeal carcinoma patients were compared. As shown in Table 4, the "highly tumorigenic" LMP1^{China1} variant was detected in 2 of 22 (9.1%) tumour samples and was absent in blood and throat lavage samples. However, as it turned out, this LMP1 variant was more common in tumour (35.7%, 5/14), blood (66.7%, 8/12) and oropharyngeal lavage (33.3%, 3/9) samples from OTOC patients, and was even detectable in one of the blood donor samples. Another LMP1^{Med+} variant, like the LMP1^{China1} variant with the 10 aa deletion, although it was detected more frequently in nasopharyngeal carcinoma specimens (tumours - 36.4% (8/22); blood 13.3% (2/15); throat lavage 31.6% (6/19)), it was also found in specimens of patients with other tumours of the oral cavity (tumours 21.4% (3/14); blood 8.3% (1/12); throat lavage 11.1% (1/9)); the differences between the corresponding values were not statistically significant.

Table 4. Multiple EBV infections and the search for tumour-specific LMP1 variants in NPC patients[1]

№	Patients' code	Tumor biopsies	Blood lymphocytes	Oropharyngeal lavages (OL)
	Nasopharyngeal carcinoma patients			
LMP1 variants in blood and/or OL samples coinciding with those in tumor samples				
1	M2	B95.8/A	B95.8/A	B95.8/A
2	M23	B95.8/A	B95.8/A	B95.8/A
3	M27	Med+	n.a.[2]	Med+
4	M28	Med+	Med+	Med+
5	M33	Med+	n.a.	Med+
6	M37	Med-	Med-	Med-
7	Lg115	B95.8/A	n.a.	B95.8/A
LMP1 variants in blood and/or OL samples not coinciding with those in tumor samples				
8	M5	OC	n.a.	Med+
9	M6	B95.8/A	NC	NC
10	M7	Med+	Med-	Med-
11	M8	Ch.1	B95.8/A	Med-
12	M11	NC	Med-	n.a.
13	M12	Med-	Med-	NC
14	M16	Med+	n.a.	B95.8/A
15	M20	Med-	NC	n.a.
16	M29	Med+	Med-	Med+
17	M42	Med+	Med-	Med+
18	M49	OC	Med+	Med-
19	Lg116	Ch.1	n.a.	B95.8/A
20	Lg117	Med+	n.a.	B95.8/A
21	Lg127	B95.8/A	OC	n.a.
22	M47	B95.8/A	B95.8/A	OC

Table 4. (Continued)

Patients with other tumors of oral cavity				
№	Patients' code	Tumor biopsies	Blood lymphocytes	Oropharyngeal lavages (OL)
LMP1 variants in blood and/or OL samples coinciding with those in tumor samples				
1	M1	Med+	n.a.	Med-
2	M25	B95.8/A	n.a.	B95.8/A
3	M32	Med+	Med+	Med+
4	M36	Med-	Med-	n.a.
5	M39	Med-	n.a.	Med-
6	M52	Ch.1	Ch.1	Ch.1
7	M54	Ch.1	Ch.1	n.a.
8	M55	Ch.1	n.a.	Ch.1
9	M56	Ch.1	Ch.1	n.a.
10	M57	Ch.1	Ch.1	n.a.
LMP1 variants in blood and/or OL samples not coinciding with those in tumor samples				
11	M18	B95.8/A	Ch.1	n.a.
12	M58	NC	Ch.1	Ch.1
13	M 1	Med +	n.a.	Med -

[1] - the data obtained demonstrate a wide variety of LMP1 variants in NPC patients compared with OTOC patients indicating the lack of tumour-specific variants in NPC patients.

[2] n.a. - no sample was available.

NPC - patients with nasopharyngeal carcinoma; OTOC - patients with other tumours of the oral cavity.

Taken together, these data, in line with results obtained by other investigators, indicate the absence of LMP1 variants specifically associated with NPC in Russia.

Amino Acid Substitutions in LMP1 Samples

Continuing the search for structural differences between EBV strains persisting in NPC and OTOC patients, LMP1 samples isolated from the tumour, blood and oropharyngeal lavage samples from both patient groups were analysed for the frequency of aa substitutions (Table 5). The data were analysed by Student's t-test.

As a result, there was no statistically significant difference in the respective values between LMP1 samples that originated from tumour and oropharyngeal lavage samples from NPC patients and those from OTOC patients (P=0.92 and P=0.32, respectively), pointing again to the genetic similarity of EBV strains that persisted in both patient groups. Higher levels of aa substitutions detected in LMP1 samples derived from the blood samples of NPC patients than from the blood samples of OTOC patients (P=0.05), could be explained by a genetic predisposition of B lymphocytes in NPC patients (due to specific HLA epitopes) to enhanced replication of EBV accompanied by mutations in the viral genome [18].

Table 5. Comparative analysis of the most frequently detected aa substitutions in LMP1 isolates from NPC patients versus patients with OTOC

№	Amino acid positions in strain $LMP1^{B95.8}$ and its substitutions	Source of LMP1 samples, patient's groups					
		Tumor biopsies		Blood samples		Oropharyngeal lavages	
		NPC n=22	OTOC n=14	NPC n=15	OTOC n=12	NPC n=19	OTOC n=9
1	229 S→T	6 (27.2%)	5 (35. %)	8 (53.3%)	2 (17.0%)	10(52.6%)	1(11.1%)
2	252 G→A	5 (22.7%)	3 (21.4%)	6 (40.0%)	0	5 (26.3%)	1 (11.1%)
3	266 D→G	6 (27.2%)	2 (14.2%)	3 (20.0%)	0	7 (36.8%)	0
4	282 D→G	6 (27.2%)	2 (14.2%)	4 (26.6%)	1 (8.3%)	7 (36.8%)	0
5	293 D→G/H	7 (31.8%)	2 (14.2%)	8 (53.3%)	1 (8.3%)	8 (42.1%)	1 (11.1%)
6	309 S→N	11(50.0%)	11(78.5%)	11 (73.3%)	10.(83.0%)	12(63.1%)	5 (55.5%)
7	317 D→N/E	8 (36.3%)	1 (7.1%)	1 (6.6%)	0	3 (15.7%)	0
8	322 Q→E/T/N/D	13 (59.0%)	13(92.8%)	9 (60.0%)	11 (92.0%)	12(63.1%)	7 (77.7%)
9	328 E→Q/A/L	6 (27.2%)	4 (28.5%)	3 (20.0%)	2 (17.0%)	2 (10.5%)	1(11.1%)
10	331 G→Q	1 (4.5%)	1 (7.1%)	2 (13.3%)	1 (8.3%)	2 (10.5%)	2 (22.2%)
11	334 Q→R	6 (27.2%)	8 (57.1%)	9 (60.0%)	8 (67%)	7 (36.8%)	3 (33.3%)
12	338 L→S/P	7 (31.8%)	11(78.5%)	9 (60.0%)	7 (58.0%)	4 (21.0%)	5 (55.5%)
13	352 H→R/N/S	5 (22.7%)	4 (28.5%)	6 (40.0%)	2 (17.0%)	8 (42.1%)	0
14	366 S→T	13 (59.0%)	14 (100%)	11(73.3%)	12 (100%)	10 (52.6)	9 (100%)
15	366 S→A	9 (40.9%)	0	4 (26.6%)	0	9 (47.4%)	0
	Means values and standard errors	36.40 (5.74)a	39.04 (8.56)	46.43 (6.60)	33.93 (9.98)	41.26 (6.35)	30.36 (9.15)
	P-value of the T-test for percent	**0.627[a]**		**0.054**		**0.145**	

Means, standard errors and P-values according to Student's T-test for frequencies of the most frequently encountered amino acid (aa) substitutions (aa positions 229–366) in LMP1 variants originating from tumor, blood and oropharyngeal lavage samples of NPC patients versus patients with OTOC are presented in the Table.

NPC - patients with nasopharyngeal carcinoma patients; OTOC - patients with other tumours of the oral cavity.

Conclusion

To date, the mechanism of EBV-associated carcinogenesis leading to NPC development remains obscure. The ubiquitous spread of the virus and varying incidence of EBV-related tumours in different geographic regions raises the possibility of the existence of particular EBV strains contributing to the development of certain EBV-associated malignancies. In the present study, carried out in a non-endemic region for nasopharyngeal carcinoma, Russia, the EBV strain with a specific LMP1 allele characteristic for NPC was not detected.

However, according to some publications, several specific EBV gene variants (the f variant, having an extra BamHI site in the BamHI F fragment, f/V29A/SPM or V-val subtype of EBNA 1), were found to be strongly associated with endemic NPC but not with other EBV-associated diseases [43-46].

The validity of this phenomenon for NPC in non-endemic regions would indicate the universality of the association between this tumour and specific EBV genes and their possible dominant role in NPC development, regardless of geographic area.

Summarising the data, this investigation carried out in Russia, which is a non-NPC endemic region, demonstrated similarity in the genetic structure of the LMP1 gene in EBV strains persisting in NPC and OTOC patients. The results of this study allow us to assume that the origin of EBV-associated pathologies will likely not link to a specific strain of EBV or its LMP1oncogene.

Any strain of the virus with any structure of LMP1 is probably capable of initiating the tumour development process, but the oncogenic potential of the virus can occur only in the case of additional human exposure to harmful factors in the internal and external environment, such as chemical carcinogens, congenital or acquired immunodeficiency, a genetic predisposition to the development of tumours and other factors. Further investigations with a larger number of observations and new methodological approaches could probably confirm or reject our suggestion and thus contribute to the understanding of the mechanism of EBV-associated carcinogenesis in non-endemic regions.

Supporting Information

With the kind permission of the Pleiades Publishing, Inc. Tables 1 and 2 with a new modifications were taken from the article "Sequence Variants of LMP1 Oncogene in Patients with Oral Cavity Tumors Associated and not associated with Epstain-Barr Virus" originally published by V. E. Gurtsevitch, L. S. Yakovleva, L. N. Scherbak, E. V. Goncharova, K. V. Smirnova, S. V. Diduk, V. N. Kondratova, D. M. Maksimovich, A. V. Lichtenstein, and N. B. Senyuta in the Molecular Biology 2013,V47, #6, pp. 863- 870.

With the kind permission of the John Wiley & Sons, Inc. Tables 3, 4, 5 and Figure 3 with minor modifications were taken from the article "Epstein–Barr Virus Latent Membrane Protein 1 Polymorphism in Nasopharyngeal Carcinoma and Other Oral Cavity Tumors in Russia" originally published by Natalia Senyuta, Larissa Yakovleva, Elena Goncharova, Liana Scherback, Sergey Diduk, Ksenia Smirnova, Dmitry Maksimovich, and Vladimir Gurtsevitch in Journal of Medical Virology 86:290–300 (2014).

Acknowledgment

We are grateful to Professors A. Mudunov, M. Kropotov, B. Poddubny, N. Probatova, N. Kondratieva, N. Mikhailova and Dr. S. Djabbarov (Institute of Clinical Oncology, FSBI N.N. Blokhin Cancer Research Center RAMS) for collection of clinical specimens from NPC and OTOC patients, the verification of diagnosis and management of the patients.

This work was supported by grant from the Russian Research Foundation (RFBI) № 13-04-00063 and by the National Program "Life Science" with subdirection "Genomic, proteomic and post-genomic technologies" № 01 200 960 425 (code of the investigation 386).

References

[1] Young L. S., Rickinson A. B. (2004). Epstein-Barr virus: 40 years on. *Nat. Rev. Cancer*, 4, 757-768.

[2] Lanier A., Bender T., Talbot M. et al. (1980). Nasopharyngeal carcinoma in Alaskan Eskimos Indians, and Aleuts: a review of cases and study of Epstein-Barr virus, HLA, and environmental risk factors. *Cancer,* 46, 2100-2106.

[3] Yu M. C. (1991). Nasopharyngeal carcinoma: epidemiology and dietary factors. *IARC Sci. Publ.*, 39-47.

[4] Yu M. C., Yuan J. M. (2002). Epidemiology of nasopharyngeal carcinoma. *Semin. Cancer Biol.*, 12, 421-429.

[5] Young L. S., Dawson C. W., Eliopoulos A. G. (2000). The expression and function of Epstein-Barr virus encoded latent genes. *Mol. Pathol.,* 53, 238-247.

[6] Abbot S. D., Rowe M., Cadwallader K. et al. (1990). Epstein-Barr virus nuclear antigen 2 induces expression of the virus-encoded latent membrane protein. *J. Virol.*, 64, 2126-2134.

[7] Li H. P., Chang Y. S. (2003). Epstein-Barr virus latent membrane protein 1: structure and functions. *J. Biomed. Sci.*, 10, 490-504.

[8] Kung C. P., Raab-Traub N. (2010). Epstein-Barr virus latent membrane protein 1 modulates distinctive NF- kappaB pathways through C-terminus-activating region 1 to regulate epidermal growth factor receptor expression. *J. Virol.*, 84, 6605-6614.

[9] Wu L., Nakano H., Wu Z. (2006). The C-terminal activating region 2 of the Epstein-Barr virus-encoded latent membrane protein 1 activates NF-kappaB through TRAF6 and TAK1. *J. Biol. Chem.*, 281, 2162-2169.

[10] Tsao S. W., Tramoutanis G., Dawson C. W. et al. (2002). The significance of LMP1 expression in nasopharyngeal carcinoma. *Semin. Cancer Biol.*, 12, 473-487.

[11] Zheng H., Li L. L., Hu D. S. et al. (2007). Role of Epstein-Barr virus encoded latent membrane protein 1 in the carcinogenesis of nasopharyngeal carcinoma. *Cell Mol. Immunol.*, 4, 185-196.

[12] Wang D., Liebowitz D., Kieff E. (1985). An EBV membrane protein expressed in immortalized lymphocytes transforms established rodent cells. *Cell*, 43, 831-840.

[13] Hu L. F., Zabarovsky E. R., Chen F. et al. (1991). Isolation and sequencing of the Epstein-Barr virus BNLF-1 gene (LMP1) from a Chinese nasopharyngeal carcinoma. *J. Gen. Virol.*, 72 (Pt 10), 2399-2409.

[14] Chen M. L., Tsai C. N., Liang C. L. et al. (1992). Cloning and characterization of the latent membrane protein (LMP) of a specific Epstein-Barr virus variant derived from the nasopharyngeal carcinoma in the Taiwanese population. *Oncogene,* 7, 2131-2140.

[15] Hu L.F., Chen F., Zheng X. et al. (1993). Clonability and tumorigenicity of human epithelial cells expressing the EBV encoded membrane protein LMP1. *Oncogene,* 8, 1575-1583.

[16] Miller W. E., Cheshire J. L., Baldwin A. S., Jr. et al. (1998). The NPC derived C15 LMP1 protein confers enhanced activation of NF-kappa B and induction of the EGFR in epithelial cells. *Oncogene,* 16, 1869-1877.

[17] Edwards R. H., Seillier-Moiseiwitsch F., Raab-Traub N. (1999). Signature amino acid changes in latent membrane protein 1 distinguish Epstein-Barr virus strains. *Virology,* 261, 79-95.

[18] Edwards R. H., Sitki-Green D., Moore D. T. et al. (2004). Potential selection of LMP1 variants in nasopharyngeal carcinoma. *J. Virol.*, 78, 868-881.

[19] Sandvej K., Gratama J. W., Munch M. et al. (1997). Sequence analysis of the Epstein-Barr virus (EBV) latent membrane protein-1 gene and promoter region: identification of four variants among wild-type EBV isolates. *Blood,* 90, 323-330.

[20] Walling D. M., Shebib N., Weaver S. C. et al. (1999). The molecular epidemiology and evolution of Epstein-Barr virus: sequence variation and genetic recombination in the latent membrane protein-1 gene. *J. Infect. Dis.,* 179, 763-774.

[21] Hahn P., Novikova E., Scherback L. et al. (2001). The LMP1 gene isolated from Russian nasopharyngeal carcinoma has no 30-bp deletion. *Int. J. Cancer*, 91, 815-821.

[22] Lawrence J. B., Villnave C. A., Singer R. H. (1988). Sensitive, high-resolution chromatin and chromosome mapping in situ: presence and orientation of two closely integrated copies of EBV in a lymphoma line. *Cell,* 52, 51-61.

[23] Lo Y. M., Chan L. Y., Lo K. W. et al. (1999). Quantitative analysis of cell-free Epstein-Barr virus DNA in plasma of patients with nasopharyngeal carcinoma. *Cancer Res.,* 59, 1188-1191.

[24] Botezatu I. V., Kondratova V. N., Shelepov V. P. et al. (2011). DNA melting analysis: application of the "open tube" format for detection of mutant KRAS. *Anal. Biochem.*, 419, 302-308.

[25] Gurtsevitch V., Ruiz R., Stepina V. et al. (1986). Epstein-Barr viral serology in nasopharyngeal carcinoma patients in the USSR and Cuba, and its value for differential diagnosis of the disease. *Int. J. Cancer*, 37, 375-381.

[26] Jo S. A., Hwang S. H., Kim S. Y. et al. (2010). Quantitation of whole blood Epstein-Barr virus DNA is useful for assessing treatment response in patients with non-Hodgkin's lymphoma. *Int. J. Lab. Hematol.*, 32, e106-e113.

[27] Lay M. L., Lucas R. M., Ratnamohan M. et al. (2010). Measurement of Epstein-Barr virus DNA load using a novel quantification standard containing two EBV DNA targets and SYBR Green I dye. *Virol. J.,* 7, 252-.

[28] Lee C. H., Yeh T. H., Lai H. C. et al. (2011). Epstein-Barr virus Zta-induced immunomodulators from nasopharyngeal carcinoma cells upregulate interleukin-10 production from monocytes. *J. Virol.*, 85, 7333-7342.

[29] Zhang G., Tsang C. M., Deng W. et al. (2013). Enhanced IL-6/IL-6R signaling promotes growth and malignant properties in EBV-infected premalignant and cancerous nasopharyngeal epithelial cells. PLoS One, 8, e62284-

[30] Trammell R. A., Verhulst S., Toth L. A. (2013). Environmental perturbation, inflammation and behavior in healthy and virus-infected mice. *Brain Behav. Immun.*, 33, 139-152.

[31] Li S. N., Chang Y. S., Liu S. T. (1996). Effect of a 10-amino acid deletion on the oncogenic activity of latent membrane protein 1 of Epstein-Barr virus. *Oncogene*, 12, 2129-2135.

[32] Miller W. E., Edwards R. H., Walling D. M. et al. (1994). Sequence variation in the Epstein-Barr virus latent membrane protein 1. *J. Gen. Virol.,* 75 (Pt 10), 2729-2740.

[33] Nagamine M., Takahara M., Kishibe K. et al. (2007). Sequence variations of Epstein-Barr virus LMP1 gene in nasal NK/T-cell lymphoma. *Virus Genes*, 34, 47-54.

[34] Efron B., Halloran E., Holmes S. (1996). Bootstrap confidence levels for phylogenetic trees. *Proc. Natl. Acad. Sci. U.S.A.,* 93, 13429-13434.

[35] Kanai K., Satoh Y., Saiki Y. et al. (2007). Difference of Epstein-Barr virus isolates from Japanese patients and African Burkitt's lymphoma cell lines based on the sequence of latent membrane protein 1. *Virus Genes,* 34, 55-61.

[36] Burrows J. M., Khanna R., Sculley T. B. et al. (1996). Identification of a naturally occurring recombinant Epstein-Barr virus isolate from New Guinea that encodes both type 1 and type 2 nuclear antigen sequences. *J. Virol.,* 70, 4829-4833.

[37] Walling D. M., Raab-Traub N. (1994). Epstein-Barr virus intrastrain recombination in oral hairy leukoplakia. *J. Virol.*, 68, 7909-7917.

[38] Sitki-Green D., Covington M., Raab-Traub N. (2003). Compartmentalization and transmission of multiple epstein-barr virus strains in asymptomatic carriers. *J. Virol.,* 77, 1840-1847.

[39] Tierney R. J., Edwards R. H., Sitki-Green D. et al. (2006). Multiple Epstein-Barr virus strains in patients with infectious mononucleosis: comparison of ex vivo samples with in vitro isolates by use of heteroduplex tracking assays. *J. Infect. Dis.,* 193, 287-297.

[40] Tierney R. J., Kao K. Y., Nagra J. K. et al. (2011). Epstein-Barr virus BamHI W repeat number limits EBNA2/EBNA-LP coexpression in newly infected B cells and the efficiency of B-cell transformation: a rationale for the multiple W repeats in wild-type virus strains. *J. Virol.,* 85, 12362-12375.

[41] Deng W., Pang P. S., Tsang C. M. et al. (2012). Epstein-Barr virus-encoded latent membrane protein 1 impairs G2 checkpoint in human nasopharyngeal epithelial cells through defective Chk1 activation. *PLoS One*, 7, e39095-

[42] Lo K. W., Chung G. T., To K. F. (2012). Deciphering the molecular genetic basis of NPC through molecular, cytogenetic, and epigenetic approaches. *Semin. Cancer Biol.,* 22, 79-86.

[43] Li J., Qian C. N., Zeng Y. X. (2009). Regulatory T cells and EBV associated malignancies. *Int. Immunopharmacol*., 9, 590-592.

[44] Lung M. L., Lam W. P., Sham J. et al. (1991). Detection and prevalence of the "f" variant of Epstein-Barr virus in southern China. *Virology,* 185, 67-71.

[45] Wang Y., Wang X. F., Sun Z. F. et al. (2012). Unique variations of Epstein-Barr virus-encoded BARF1 gene in nasopharyngeal carcinoma biopsies. *Virus Res.,* 166, 23-30.

[46] Zhang X. S., Wang H. H., Hu L. F. et al. (2004). V-val subtype of Epstein-Barr virus nuclear antigen 1 preferentially exists in biopsies of nasopharyngeal carcinoma. *Cancer Lett.,* 211, 11-18.

In: Head and Neck Cancer
Editor: Madison R. Hall
ISBN: 978-1-63482-113-1

Chapter 7

Side Effects of Cetuximab Rash

Ana Cvetanovic*[*1], Sladjana Filipovic[1,2], Svetislav Vrbic[1,2], Ivica Pejcic[1,2] and Lazar Popovic[3,4]
[1]Medical Oncology Unit, University Clinic Nis, Serbia
[2]Oncology at Medical Faculty, University of Nis, Serbia
[3]Oncology Institute of Vojvodina, Serbia
[4]Oncology at Medical Faculty,
University of Novi Sad, Serbia

Abstract

The use of epidermal growth factor receptor (EGFR) inhibitors in several types of cancer has increased considerably in recent years. Currently they are approved in non-small cell lung cancer (NSCLC), pancreatic cancer, colorectal cancer (CRC) and squamous-cell carcinoma of the head and neck (SCCHN). Monoclonal antibodies against the EGFR (cetuximab, panitumumab) or EGFR tyrosine kinase inhibitors (gefitinib, erlotinib, lapatinib) are generally well tolerated and do not have the severe systemic side effect usually seen with cytotoxic drugs. A considerable number of patients treated with these EGFR inhibitors, however, develop dermatological side-effects, most frequently a papulopustular rash but also eczema, xerosis, telangiectasia, hyper-pigmentation, fissures, paronychia and hair changes. EGFR is normally expressed in the basal layer of the epidermis and contributes of the stimulation of epidermal growth, inhibition of differentiation and acceleration of wound healing. Inhibition of EGFR results in impaired growth, migration of keratinocytes, inflammatory chemokine expression of these cells and subsequent cutaneous injury. Desruption of these barrier may also promote bacterial overgrowth, further exarcebating injury to the cutaneous tissue.

Cetuximab related -skin toxicity have been reported in 60%-80% in patients with mCRC treated with cetuximab monotherapy with a similar frequency seen in trials of cetuximab in combination with chemotherapy. The most common adverse events among patients treated with cetuximab is the papulopustular rash. The onset of rash is

* Corresponding author: Dr Ana Cvetanovic, MD, Medical oncology unit, University Clinic Nis, Serbia, ana.stankovic@yahoo.com

early,generally developing over a period of six weeks after starting treatment. Incidencs and severity are usually dose dependent.

Effective and timing treatment of cetuximab related rash is mandatory to maximize the anti-tumor efficacy of cetuximab as well as maintaining the patients quality of life. Mild cases respond well to topical anti-infammatory therapy whereas tetracyclines and corticosteroids are needed to treat moderate to severe cases.

Available data suggests that the appearance and severity of skin rash is positively correlated with objective tumor response to cetuximab therapy and with overall survival. Data suggest that skin rash may serve as a surrogate marker of EGFR-targeted mAb efficacy. In patients receiving cetuximab monotherapy for refractory mCRC, longer survival times were observed in patients with rash of any grade as compared with patients experiencing no rash ($p = 0.02$).

In the BOND trial of cetuximab in combination with irinotecan as compared with cetuximab alone in patients with mCRC, response rates in patients with skin reaction were higher than rates in patients without skin reaction (25.8% vs. 6.3% in the combination group, 13.0% vs. 0% in the monotherapy group; $p = 0.005$).

Data from the CRYSTAL trial support this observation as the median PFS of patients without rash was 5,4 months compared to 9,4 months in patients with grade 2 and 11.3 in patients with grade 3 toxicity. The phase I/II of EVEREST study showed that response rate and skin toxicity both increased with dose excalation.

The introduction of cetuximab in colorectal and head and neck cancer therapy had a significant impact on outcomes. A strategic approach to the management of skin toxicity will allow one to limit the incidence of skin rash, to improve patients` compliance and to optimize outcomes.

Introduction

The epidermal growth factor receptor (EGFR, HER1, erbB1) is a 170-kDa protein made of three domain:an extracellular ligand-binding domain, a short transmembrane domain, and an intracellular domain with intrinsic tyrosine kinase activity. Overexpression or hyperactivity of the EGFR has been shown to play a leading role in the progression of several epithelial neoplasms [1, 2]. The EGFR is activated by binding of ligand to its extracellular domain which leads to receptor homodimerization or heterodimerization with any of the other three members of this family of transmembrane tyrosine kinases: HER2 (erbB2), HER3 (erbB3), and HER4 (erbB4). This results in binding of ATP to the receptor's catalytic site followed by activation of the receptor's tyrosine kinase and autophosphorylation on C-terminal tyrosine residues, which, in turn, recruit several cytoplasmic signal transducers. These effector molecules include PLC-italic gamma1, Ras-MEK-MAPK, phosphatidylinositol-3 kinase (PI3K) and its target Akt, p70S6 kinase, Src, STATs, and others [2, 3].

The oncogenic potential of the EGFR and its high level of expression in tumor tissues provides a reason for targeting this oncoprotein with novel molecular therapeutic agents. Indeed, anti-EGFR molecules inhibit the progression of EGFR-dependent preclinical models and have recently demonstrated clinical efficacy against several human carcinomas [4]. The antitumor effect of these inhibitors requires the subversion of key postreceptor signaling pathways and cell cycle/apoptosis regulatory molecules that mediate the transforming effects of the EGFR network. Inactivation of constitutively active MAPK and the serine/threonine kinase Akt, a target of PI3K, have been reported in EGFR-dependent tumor cells treated with EGFR inhibitors [5, 6, 7, 8, 9].

The human epidermal growth factor receptor (HER1/EGFR) is a transmembrane glycoprotein of the tyrosine kinase growth factor family that is expressed in many normal human tissues. It is finely regulated to control cell growth and proliferation. In many cancers, this growth factor is dysregulated and overexpressed, and this overexpression is common in many solid tumors, such as colorectal (65-75%), head and neck (90%), and lung (60%-90%) carcinomas. It is linked with increased metastasis, reduced survival, and a poor prognosis [10].

Overexpression can result in uncontrolled cell growth, proliferation, angiogenesis and metastases. This growth factor can be successfully blocked by antibodies against the extracellular domain of the receptor, or small molecule inhibitors directed against the intracellular tyrosine kinase domain and most of the EGFR inhibitors can be classified into two categories: monoclonal antibodies and tyrosine kinase inhibitors. Numerous EGFR inhibitors are under development, but to date only five of them are FDA-approved, including three that inhibit the receptor's intracellular tyrosine kinase activity (gefitinib, erlotinib and lapatinib) and two that block extracellular ligand binding (cetuximab and panitumumab) [11].

Cetuximab, in particular, also inhibits the production of angiogenic factors, mediates antibody-dependent cell-mediated cytotoxicity, and works synergistically with chemotherapy and radiotherapy [12, 13]. Cetuximab (IMC- C225, Erbitux, ImClone Systems/Bristol-Myers Squibb), a chimeric human/murine monoclonal antibody, has been approved by the Food and Drug Administration (FDA) on july 6 2012, for the treatment of EGFR-positive metastatic colorectal carcinoma (CRC) in patients who are intolerant to irinotecan-based chemotherapy as well as in combination with irinotecan in patients who are refractory to irinotecan-based chemotherapy . This approval was based on retrospective analyses of tumor samples from patients enrolled in the CRYSTAL trial and in two supportive studies, CA225025 and EMR 62 202-047 (OPUS), according to K-ras mutation status. The addition of cetuximab to chemotherapy or best supportive care (BSC) resulted in improved survival (OS), progression-free survival (PFS), and overall responses rate (ORR) in patients with K-ras wild-type tumors, whereas there was no benefit, or even potential harm, in patients with K-ras mutant tumors.

In addition, cetuximab was approved by the FDA in March 2006 for the treatment of recurrent or metastatic squamous cell carcinoma of the head and neck (SCCHN) in patients who are not responsive to platinum-based chemotherapy, as well as locally or regionally advanced SCCHN when used in combination with radiation therapy [14]. It has also been evaluated for non-small-cell lung cancer (NSCLC), renal cell carcinoma, and advanced pancreatic cancer [15-17].

The major side effect associated with cetuximab treatment is skin toxicity, including skin rash, dry skin, hair growth disorders, pruritus, and nail changes [18, 19]. Although the skin toxicities are usually not dose-limiting or lethal, they can cause patients significant physical and psychosocial discomfort that impair on treatment adherence and clinical outcomes of EGFR inhibitors. Therefore, appropriate management is necessary to allow acceptable drug administration and to improve health-related quality of life and outcomes.

Interest in rash has recently increased because it was suggested to have a possible relationship with clinical outcomes [20-22]. Interestingly, a positive association between the presence and severity of EGFR inhibitor-associated-skin rash and tumor response and survival has been consistently observed with all EGFR inhibitors approved for clinical use

.These findings suggest that skin toxicity may be a useful surrogate marker of successful EGFR inhibition in the tumors and clinical benefit from the EGFR inhibitors. Increasing attention has been drawn to understand the mechanism and improve the management of skin toxicities to EGFR inhibitors, especially skin rash [23-24].

Pathophysiology of Cetuximab-Induced Skin Rash EGFR Expression in the Skin

Normal skin is composed of three layers: the epidermis-the most superficial layer, the dermis which providing support and tensile strength, and the hypodermis -adipose tissue. The basal layer of the skin is contiguous with the outer root sheath of the hair follicle, sharing biochemical properties and high EGFR expression, which are essential to maintain the homeostasis of their structural integrity and function [25- 27]. The epidermis is predominantly made of keratinocytes, which undergo a highly regulated process of differentiation and migration nearly the skin surface and the outer layers of the hair follicle. EGFR is primarily expressed in undifferentiated, proliferating keratinocytes in the basal and suprabasal layers of the epidermis. EGFR signaling activates epidermal growth and differentiation, accelerates wound healing and stimulates vasoconstriction and keratinocyte migration. Expression of EGFR is lost as keratinocytes exit the basal layer, a process that is characterized by growth arrest and initiation of differentiation [28,29]. High level of EGFR is also expressed in sebaceous epithelium, eccrine epithelium, dendritic antigen-presenting cells and various connective tissues. Activation of EGFR by its ligands, mainly TGF alpha and heparin-binding EGF in the skin, has been shown to regulate normal keratinocyte proliferation, differentiation, migration and survival via downstream signal transduction cascades, mainly the MAPK pathway, the PI3K/Akt pathway, and the Jak/STAT pathway [27, 29].

Consistent with the high-density distribution of sebaceous glands, skin rash occurs most commonly in the scalp, face, and upper chest, where high levels of EGFR expression are present. EGFR inhibitors can have several effects on epithelial homeostasis like abnormal maturation and skin differentiation, growth and migration arrest, an increased rate of apoptosis and an inflammatory response leading to tissue damage and skin atrophy. Severe acute skin reactions show massive neutrophilic infiltration of the epidermis and, extreme apoptosis.

This result in a sensory disturbance and papulopustular rash within the first few days or weeks of therapy. Chronic skin changes are characterized by epidermal atrophy, disappearance of follicular structures and epidermal fissures [28]. Maturation and differentiation are also impaired, and these changes will become evident later on, when xerosis and nail and hair growth disturbances predominate. In summary, EGFR inhibitor treatment induces a complex pattern of tissue injury and inflammatory cell recruitment, damaging the basal epidermis, the sweat and sebaceous glands and hair follicles. [27].

Clinical Findings

The most common adverse event among patients treated with Cetuximab is the acneiform rash, characterized by erythematous inter and intrafollicular papulopustules and commonly affecting sun exposed areas of the body such as face, neck, shoulders, upper body and scalp. The eruption is usually confined to seborrheic areas but sometimes it may involve the extremities, lower back, abdomen, and buttocks [30, 31]. Lesions may consolidate into plaques covered with pustules that dry and form yellow crusts. Rarely an edematous, warm erythema of the face, sometimes with follicular papulo-pustules and telangiectasia resembling rosacea, is seen. In contrast to acneiform eruptions caused by other drugs, the rash may be accompanied by pruritus which sometimes can be severe. Cultures are negative for yeasts and bacteria. Papulo-pustular lesion may become infected, usually with Staphylococcus aureus then, oozing and yellowish crusts occur [32, 33].

The onset of rash is early, developing over a period of six weeks after starting treatment with Cetuximab. The first week is characterized by erythema, sensory disturbance and oedema.These symptoms are consistent with initial inhibition of EGFR in basal keratinocytes, which causing the recruitment of leukocytes, vascular dilatation and increased permeability [34].

During the second week papulo-pustular eruption appears, consist of increased numbers of inflammatory cells and debris in the superfitial layer, accompanied by varying degrees of oedema and vasodilatation.The folliculocentric nature of the rash can be explained by a larger number of affected EGFR-bearing keratinocytes per unit area in the follicle. The frequent localization of the papulopustules to the scalp, face and upper body reflect an increased density of follicles in this area [35].

The crusting stage appears by week four. The formation of crusts and the presence of neutrophils, as well as the lesions being negative for bacterial growth and rapid resolution of the rash following epidermal growth factor receptor inhibitor (EGFRI) discontinuation, supports the idea that the crusts arise because of EGFRI treatment and not as a result of an opportunistic infection. The rash is reversible, usually with complete resolution within 4 weeks of treatment discontinuation or sometimes during continued treatment but it may relapse or worsen at treatment restart. With long-term treatment, severity of rash may decrease. In some cases the rash may improve spontaneously [32, 36].

Incidence and severity is usually dose-dependent which showed in phase I escalation study [32, 37, 38].

Grading System

The most commonly used grading system for skin toxicity is the National Cancer Institute Common Terminology Criteria for Adverse Events version 4.0 (NCI CTCAE v 4.0) [39]:

Grade 1- Papules and/or pustules covering <10% BSA, which may or may not be associated with symptoms of pruritus or tenderness

Table 1. Frequency of skin toxicity in Phase II/III studies evaluating Cetuximab mono- and combination therapy in mCRC, SCCHN and NSCLC

Study	Treatment arms	n	Any grade	P value	Grade 3 or higher	P value
CRC						
CAIRO 2 study[43]	CAPOX/Bev and CET CAPOX/Bev	366 366			25% <1%	<0.01
EPIC study [44]	Irinotecan and cetuximab Irinotecan	638 629	76% 5%	<0.05	8% <1%	<0.05
Jonker et al.[45]	BSC and cetuximab BSC	288 274	89% 16%	<0.01	12% <1%	<0.01
CRYSTAL study [46]	FOLFIRI and cetuximab FOLFIRI	600 602	NR NR	--	20% <1%	<0.01
BOND study [47]	Irinotecan and cetuximab Cetuximab	218 111	80% 80%		9.4% 5.2%	<0.20
OPUS study [48]	FOLFOX 4 and Cetuximab FOLFOX 4	169 168	NR NR	--	11% <1%	<0.05
BOND 2 study [49]	Irinotecan and CET and BEV CET and BEV	43 40	83% 85%		21% 20%	
SCCHN						
Bonner et al.[50]	Radiotherapy and CET Radiotherapy	208 212	87% 10%	<0.01	17% 1%	<0.01
Vermorken et.[51]	Platinum/fluorouracil and CET Platinum/fluorouracil	219 215	NR NR	--	9% <1%	<0.01
Burtness et al.[52]	Cisplatin and cetuximab Cisplatin	58 58	77% 24%	<0.01	23% 0	NR
NSCLC						
Lynch et al. [53]	Taxane/carboplatin and CET Taxane/carboplatin	325 320	NR NR	--	11% 0	NR
FLEX study [54]	Cisplatin/vinorelbine and CET Cisplatin/vinorelbine	548 562	70% 7%	NR	10% <1%	<0.01

Abbreviations: BSC- best supportive care; CAPOX- capecitabine and oxaliplatin; FOLFIRI- fluorouracil, leucovorin, and irinotecan; FOLFOX- fluorouracil, leucovorin, and oxaliplatin; NR- not reported.

Grade 2- Papules and/or pustules covering 10 - 30% BSA, which may or may not be associated with symptoms of pruritus or tenderness; associated with psychosocial impact; limiting instrumental activities of daily living (ADL)

Grade 3-Papules and/or pustules covering >30% BSA, which may or may not be associated with symptoms of pruritus or tenderness; limiting self care ADL; associated with local superinfection with oral antibiotics indicated

Grade 4-Papules and/or pustules covering any % BSA, which may or may not be associated with symptoms of pruritus or tenderness and are associated with extensive superinfection with IV antibiotics indicated; life-threatening consequences.

This classification, however, was not specifically designed to classify cutaneous side effects of EGFRI therapy. A new version that distinguishes the diverse drug-related skin manifestations, including EGFR-i skin toxicity, has been released [39], but it is not in the practical use yet. Important factors not yet taken into consideration include the prevalent type (e.g., papular vs. pustular), the density, the total number of lesions and the infiltration of skin lesions.

Local superinfection may not always be a relevant aggravating factor. Wollenberg et al. proposed a new composite objective scoring system specific for the acneiform eruption, which considers the type of lesions and emphasizes the facial involvement, taking into account self-related symptoms [40]. Moreover, Lacouture et al. have recently presented a new grading scale specific to EGFR-i cutaneous toxicity. This grading system needs to be validated in future clinical trials [41].

In clinical trial of Cetuximab, rash occurred in the majority of patients, but in most cases is mild to moderate (Table 1.) and it is severe (grade 3 or 4) in 5%-20% of patients. In our study any degree of skin toxicity was observed in 79.41% (27/34) of the patients. Clinicaly mild to moderate skin toxicity (grade 0-2) was observed in 85 %, and grade 3 or 4 in 15 % of the patients. Grade 4 skin toxicity was documented in 1 patient [42].

Predictive Factors

There are nine reports on possible predictive factors for the occurrence and intensity of Cetuximab induced skin toxicity.

These factors may be useful to identify groups of patients who are at increased risk and who should be monitored frequently or maybe receive prophylactic treatment. Associations between age, performance score, race or skin type with an increased risk of skin toxicity have been evaluated but the results are inconsistent [55-58].

Lurje et al. was analyzing data from Cetuximab trials, reported that skin toxicity is more common in patients with a good performance score [56], whereas a study performed by Jatoi et al., evaluating 933 patients with mCRC who received.

Cetuximab, did not find such a relationship [55]. In addition, while the later study reported an association between younger age and the severity of skin toxicity, three other studies did not support this outcome [56]. Also, it is not clear yet whether race or skin color influences the occurrence and severity of skin toxicity. Factors such as polymorphisms and mutations detected in tumor tissue have been analyzed to determine their predictive value in the development of severe skin toxicity. These factors include EGFR gene copy number variants, EGFR polymorphisms and COX2 expression. Although, not much research is focused on addressing this interesting question in this moment [57, 58].

Prognostic Value of Cetuximab-Related Skin Toxicity

The positive association between the presence and severity of skin toxicity and improved tumor response and survival was first demonstrated in the phase II studies using Cetuximab in several tumors including colorectal cancer, head and neck cancer, non small cell lung cancer, pancretic and prostata cancer. Responses have been shown to correlate with the severity of the rash in phase II/III studies. In five phase II studies, patients who developed acne-like rash were shown to have longer OS. (Table 2) Skin toxicity, a well-known predictor of response, was one of the predictor variables in our data and it was in line with what was expected. When all 34 cetuximab-treated patients were analyzed, clinically relevant skin toxicity (grade 2-4) proved to be associated with significantly higher response to treatment than skin toxicity grade 0-1, with regard to ORR (80.00% vs. 20.00%), disease control rate -DCR (66.66% vs. 33.33%) and PFS (22.82 vs.12.65 weeks) [42].

The BOND trial reported higher response rates in patients with skin rash compared with patients without skin rash (25.8 vs. 6.3% respectively, p=0.005) [47]. Lenz et al. investigated 346 mCRC patients refractory to standard chemotherapy, who received CTX in a multicenter phase II trial. The median RR in the whole group was 12,4%. Patients with grade 1, 2 and 3 toxicity had a RR of 7,2%, 17% and 20%, respectively [60]. Similarly, Saltz et al. showed longer survival in patients with severe skin toxicity [20]. The analysis of this ten studies showed that the occurrence of skin rash induced by cetuximab also resulted in a statistically significant improvement in PFS,OS and response rate compared with no skin rash. Data suggest that skin rash may serve as a surrogate marker of cetuximab efficacy.

Management of Skin Rash

The skin rash from Cetuximab is transient despite of continuous treatment and is reversible after discontinuation of cetuximab. The goal of managing cetuximab related skin rash is to minimize the harmfull effects on patient` quality of life and treatment course. Optimal patient management strategies is becoming increansingly important and remains a significant area of new educational need for many clinical oncologist, oncology nurses and general practitioner [68].

Table 2. Correlation between skin toxicity with tumor response and survival

Study	Phase	Indication	Treatment	No of patients received CTX	Skin rash	PFS in patients with rash vs. patients without rash (months)	OS in patients with rash vs. patients without rash (months)	ORR in patients with rash vs. patients without rash RR
Stintzing S et al. [59]	II	mCRC	(Cetuximab+ capecitabine/irinotecan) vs. (cetuximab + capecitabine/oxaliplatin)	149	103 (69%)	7.5 vs 5.2	30 vs. 18	62%vs. 41%
Lenz et al. [60]	II	mCRC	Cetuximab monotherapy	346	311 (89%)	NR	1.7 vs 9.4	12.9% vs. O%
Boccia et al. [61]	II	mCRC	FOLFOX6 Plus Cetuximab	80	70 (87%)	NR	23 vs. 5.3	NR
Hitt et al. [62]	II	mSCCHN	Paclitaxel and cetuximab, weekly, until disease progression	46	30 (66%)	NR	NR	63% vs.37%
Maubec et al. [63]	II	Unresectable squamous cell skin cancer	Cetuximab monotherapy	36	28 (78%)	4.5 vs. 1.7.	8.9 vs. 4.0	37% vs. 0%
Fleming et al. [64]	II	Metastatic prostate cancer	(Cetuximab + mitoxantrone + prednisone) vs. (mitoxantrone + prednisone)	75	24 (32%)	10.3 vs. 2.8	21.3 vs 9.3.	8.3%vs 7.3%
Burtness et al. [65]	III	Metastatic carcinoma of the head and neck	Cisplatin every 4 weeks, with weekly cetuximab (arm A) or placebo (arm B)	57	14 (24%)	4.2 vs 2.7	9.8 vs. 8.0.	33% vs. 7%
Bonner et al. [50,66]	III	Advanced head and neck cancer	(Radiotherapy + weekly doses of cetuximab) vs. RT alone	208	204 (98%)	NR	49.0 vs 29.3	NR
Jonker et al. [45]	III	mCRC	Cetuximab + supportive care vs. supportive care alone	288	255 (88%)	NR	2.6 vs 8.4	NR
Gatzemeier et al. [67]	III	Advanced NSCLC	Chemotherapy + cetuximab vs. chemotherapy alone	518	290 (55%)	5.4 vs 4.3	15 vs. 8.8	44.8% vs 32%

Abbreviations:CTX-cetuximab, PFS-progresion free survival, OS-overall survival, ORR-overall response rate,mCRC-metastatic colorectal cancer, NR-not reported.

General Prophylactic Measures

Before the start of Cetuximab treatment full body skin evaluation should be performed. Some general interventions may be advised to patients like:

- patient should be advices to take sunscreens
- patient should be adviced to avoid activities and skin care products that dry the skin (e.g. hot water, alcohol based products..)
- enhancing skin hidration (bath oils, alcohol free moisturizing cream..)
- avoiding tight shoes
- using pre-shaving cream and moisturizing aftershave and other [69].

Skin Rash Treatment Recommendations

Grade 1

For mild reactions no dose modifications or treatment interruptions are needed. For this grade no tretament or start only with treatment with topical antibiotics like: clyndamicin 1% gel, erythromicin 3% gel or cream, metronidazole 0.75%-1% gel or cream twice daily or topical corticosteroids (hydrocortisone 2.5%, alclometasone) also twice daily.

Grade 2

No dose modification or treatment interruption are indicated. Topical antibitotics or topical corticosteroids can be used twice daily until improvements to grade 1. When papules prevail no systemic therapy recommended. When pustules prevails oral synthetic tetracycline (minocycline 100mg/day, doxycycline 100mg/day, or antibiotics covering skin flora) twice daily for at least 4 weeks is suggested, until the rash is symptomatic. In cases where secondary infections are suspected, a bacterial swab culture should be performed in order to institute oral antibiotic therapy based on sensitivities.

Grade 3

First occurrence- consider a dose interruption for 2 weeks or until the rash is grade ≤ 2. At improvement, if response to Cetuximab had been obtained continue therapy with full dose on 250 mg/m2. If no improvement occurs, discontinue therapy.

Second occurrence- delay infusion one-two weeks or until the rash is grade ≤ 2. At improvement, if response to Cetuximab had been obtained continue therapy with reduced dose on 200 mg/m2. If no improvement occurs, discontinue therapy.

Third occurrence- delay infusion one-two weeks or until the rash is grade ≤ 2. At improvement, if response to Cetuximab had been obtained continue therapy with reduced dose on 150 mg/m2. If no improvement occurs, discontinue therapy.

Fourth occurence- discontinue therapy.

In addition, oral corticosteroids (methylprednisolone 0.4 mg/kg or prednisone 0.5 mg/kg for 7 days) may be beneficial. Also for grade 3 rash, topical corticosteroids and oral antibiotics should continue upon rechallenge with EGFR inhibitors. Application of a skin moisturizer and a broad-spectrum sunscreen with an SPF of at least 30 when going outside is recommended in all patients, since the rash is accompanied by dry skin and may be aggravated by sun exposure.

For grade 3 highly symptomatic or nonresponsive patients treatment with intravenous corticosteroids (dexamethasone, methylprednisolone),oral retinoids (isotretionin 0.3-0.5 mg/kg, intravenous antihistamines, intravenous antibiotics (gentamicine or amoxicillin/clavulanic acid) and hydration can be considered.

Grade 4

Interrupt Cetuximab treatment immediately and definitely. Provide topical treatment as for grades 2 or 3. Consider systemic treatment with oral retionids, intravenous corticosteroids, intramuscular/intravenous antihistamines, intravenous antibiotics and intravenous hydration.

Prevention of acneiform rash caused by Cetuximab includes topical corticosteroids (hydrocortisone 2.5%, alclometasone) and oral antibiotics (minocycline, doxycycline, or antibiotics covering skin flora) twice daily for at least the first 6 weeks.

This results in a reduction of grade 2 and greater skin toxicities by more than 50%. In addition, these measures lessen the need to modify the dose of Cetuximab [18, 68,70-74]. Study which was done by Scope et al. Showed that prophylactic oral monicycline 100 mg daily may be useful in reducing the severity of skin rash, during the first 8 weeks of cetuximab therapy [75].

Conclusion

Increased clinical use of EGFR inhibitors has identified skin toxicity as a unique class-specific toxicity. Specific adverse skin reactions like acneiform rash occur in a large percentage of patients treated with Cetuximab. Most cases are mild to moderate and respond well to topical therapy and tetracycline antibiotics. The mechanism are poorly understood but are most likely linked to inhibition of EGFR in the skin. Cetuximab related skin rash occurs early in the course of treatment and is a potent indicator of favourable outcome. The severity of the rash is correlated with efficacy of treatment and rash may serve as a surrogate marker for tumor response.

With the increasing clinical use of EGFR inhibitors in solid tumors the optimal management of skin reactions are more than necessary. A strategic approach to the management of skin toxicity will allow one to limit the incidence of skin rash to improve patients quality of life and optimize outcomes. Despite current knowledge additional studies to better understand the mechanisms of skin toxicity and what will be effective against them are necessary.

References

[1] Prenzel N, Fischer OM, Streit S, Hart S and Ullrich A. The epidermal growth factor receptor family as a central element for cellular signal transduction and diversification. *Endocr. Relat. Cancer* 2001;8:11–31.

[2] Yarden Y and Sliwkowski MX. Untangling the ErbB signalling network. *Nat. Rev. Mol. Cell Biol.* 2001;2:127–137.

[3] Olayioye MA, Neve RM, Lane HA and Hynes NE. The ErbB signaling network: receptor heterodimerization in development and cancer *EMBO J* 2000;19:3159–3167.

[4] Arteaga CL. The epidermal growth factor receptor: from mutant oncogene in nonhuman cancers to therapeutic target in human neoplasia. *J. Clin. Oncol.* 2001:19:32S–40S.

[5] Fan Z, Shang BY, Lu Y, Chou JL and Mendelsohn J. Reciprocal changes in p27(Kip1) and p21(Cip1) in growth inhibition mediated by blockade or overstimulation of epidermal growth factor receptors. *Clin. Cancer Res.* 1997;3:1943–1948.

[6] Busse D, Doughty RS, Ramsey TT, Russell WE, Price JO, Flanagan WM, Shawver LK and Arteaga CL. Reversible G1 Arrest Induced by Inhibition of the Epidermal Growth Factor Receptor Tyrosine Kinase Requires Up-regulation of p27KIP1 Independent of MAPK Activity *J. Biol. Chem.* 2000;275:6987–6995.

[7] Lenferink AE, Busse D, Flanagan WM, Yakes FM and Arteaga CL. ErbB2/neu kinase modulates cellular p27(Kip1) and cyclin D1 through multiple signaling pathways.*Cancer Res.* 2001;61:6583–6591.

[8] Albanell J, Codony-Servat J, Rojo F, Del Campo JM, Sauleda S, Anido J, Raspall G, Giralt J, Rosello J, Nicholson RI, Mendelsohn J and Baselga J. Activated extracellular signal-regulated kinases: association with epidermal growth factor receptor /transforming growth factor alpha expression in head and neck squamous carcinoma and inhibition by anti-epidermal growth factor receptor treatments. *Cancer Res.*2001;61:6500–6510.

[9] Nelson JM and Fry DW.Akt, MAPK (Erk1/2), and p38 Act in Concert to Promote Apoptosis in Response to ErbB Receptor Family Inhibition. *J. Biol. Chem.* 2001;276:14842–14847.

[10] Salomon DS, Brandt R, Ciardiello F, Normanno N. Epidermal growth factor-related peptides and their receptors in human malignancies. *Crit Rev. Oncol. Hematol* 1995;19(3):183-232.

[11] Pinaki R.Dutta, Amit Maity. Cellular responses to EGFR inhibitors and their relevance to cancer therapy. *Cancer Letters* 2007;254(2):165–177.

[12] Harris M. Monoclonal antibodies as therapeutic agents for cancer. *Lancet Oncol.* 2004;5:292-302.

[13] Ciardiello F, Bianco R, Damiano V, Fontanini G, Caputo R, Pomatico G, et al. Antiangiogenic and antitumor activity of anti-epidermal growth factor receptor C225 monoclonal antibody in combination with vascular endothelial growth factor antisense oligonucleotide in human GEO colon cancer cells.*Clin Cancer Res* 2000;6:3739-47.

[14] Food and Drug Administration. Available from:http://www.fda.gov/cder/foi/appletter /2004/125084ltr.pdf.

[15] Bogart JA, Govindan R. A randomized phase II study of radiation therapy, pemetrexed, and carboplatin with or without cetuximab in stage III non-small-cell lung cancer. *Clin. Lung Cancer* 2006;7:285-287.

[16] Motzer RJ, Amato R, Todd M, Hwu WJ, Cohen R, Baselga J, et al. Phase II trial of antiepidermal growth factor receptor antibody C225 in patients with advanced renal cell carcinoma. *Invest New Drugs* 2003;21:99-101.

[17] Krempien R, Muenter MW, Huber PE, Nill S, Friess H, Timke C, et al. Randomized phase II study evaluating EGFR targeting therapy with cetuximab in combination with

radiotherapy and chemotherapy for patients with locally advanced pancreatic cancer - PARC: study protocol [ISRCTN56652283]. *BMC Cancer* 2005;5:131.

[18] Segaert S, Van Cutsem E. Clinical signs, pathophysiology and management of skin toxicity during therapy with epidermal growth factor receptor inhibitors. *Ann. Oncol.* 2005; 16: 1425-1433.

[19] Lacouture ME. Mechanisms of cutaneous toxicities to EGFR inhibitors. *Nat. Rev. Cancer* 2006;6:803-812.

[20] Saltz LB, Meropol NJ, Loehrer PJ, et al. Phase II trial of cetuximab in patients with refractory colorectal cancer that expresses the epidermal growth factor receptor. *J. Clin. Oncol* 2004;22:1201-1208.

[21] Bonner JA, Harari PM, Giralt J, et al. Radiotherapy plus cetuximab for locoregionally advanced head and neck cancer: 5-year survival data from a phase 3 randomised trial, and relation between cetuximab-induced rash and survival. *Lancet Oncol.* 2010;11:21-28.

[22] Vermorken JB, Mesia R, Rivera F, et al. Platinum-based chemotherapy plus cetuximab in head and neck cancer. *N. Engl. J. Med* 2008;359:1116-1127.

[23] Perez-Soler R, Saltz L. Cutaneous adverse effects with HER1/EGFR-targeted agents: is there a silver lining?. *J. Clin. Oncol* 2005;23:5235–5246.

[24] Wacker B, Nagrani T, Weinberg J et al. Correlation between development of rash and efficacy in patients treated with the epidermal growth factor receptor tyrosine kinase inhibitor erlotinib in two large phase III studies. *Clin. Cancer Res.* 2007;13:3913–3921.

[25] Lacouture ME. Mechanisms of cutaneous toxicities to EGFR inhibitors. *Nat. Rev. Cancer* 2006;6:803–812.

[26] Jost M, Kari C, Rodeck U.The EGF receptor—an essential regulator of multiple epidermal functions. *Eur. J. Dermatol* 2000;10:505–510.

[27] Woodworth CD, Michael E, Marker D et al.Inhibition of the epidermal growth factor receptor increases expression of genes that stimulate inflammation, apoptosis, and cell attachment. *Mol. Cancer Ther* 2005;4:650–658.

[28] Lacouture ME, Basti S, Patel J,Benson A 3rd. The SERIES clinic: an interdisciplinary approach to the management of toxicities of EGFR inhibitors. *J. Support Oncol.* 2006;4:236-238.

[29] Mitchell EP, Perez-Soler R, Van Cutsem E, Lacouture ME. Clinical presentation and pathophysiology of EGFRI dermatologic toxicities. Oncology (Williston Park) 2007;21:4-9.

[30] Jacot W, Bessis D, Jorda E, et al. Acneiform eruption induced by epidermal growth factor receptor inhibitors in patients with solid tumours. *Br. J. Dermatol* 2004;151(1):238-241.

[31] Bianchini D, Jayanth A, Chua YJ,et al. Epidermal growth factor receptor inhibitor-related skin toxicity:mechanism, treatments and its potential role as a predictive marker. *Clin. Colorectal. Cancer* 2008;7(1);33-43.

[32] Rowinsky EK, Schwartz GH, Gollob JA, et al. Safety, pharmacokinetics, and activity of ABX-EGF, a fully human anti-epidermal growth factor receptor monoclonal antibody in patients with metastatic renal cell cancer. *J. Clin. Oncol* 2004;22:3003-3035.

[33] Jatoi A, Green EM, Rowland KM, et al. Clinical predictors of severe cetuximab-induced rash: observations from 933 patients enrolled in north central cancer treatment group study N0147. *Oncology* 2009;77:120-123.

[34] Van Doorn R, Kirtschig G, Scheffer E, Stoof TJ, Giaccone G. Follicular and epidermal alterations in patients treated with ZD 1839(Iressa), an inhibitor of the epidermal growth factor receptor. *Br. J. Dermatol* 2002;147:598-601.

[35] Treudler R, Zouboulis CC. Follicular drug eruption induced by gefitinib (ZD 1839,Iressa):clinical picture correlates with in vitro data of focal epidermal necrosis after epidermal growth factor inhibition in skin cultures. *Int. J. Dermatol* 2005;44:167-168.

[36] Cunningham D, Humblet Y, Siena S, et al. Cetuximab monotherapy and cetuximab plus irinotecan in irinotecan-refractory metastatic colorectal cancer. *N. Engl. J. Med.* 2004;351:337-345.

[37] Hidalgo M, Siu LL, Nemunaitis J, et al. Phase I and pharmacologic study of OSI-774, an epidermal growth factor receptor tyrosine kinase inhibitor, in patients with advanced solid malignancies. *J. Clin. Oncol.* 2001;19(13):3267-3279.

[38] Foon KA, Yang XD, Weiner LM, et al. Preclinical and clinical evaluation of ABX-EGF,a fully human anti-epidermal growth factor receptor antibody. *Int. J. Radiat. Oncol. Biol. Phys.* 2004;58(3):984-990.

[39] National Cancer Institute. Common terminology criteria for adverse event v. 2.0 1999, v. 3.0 2006, v. 4.0 2009. http://ctep.cancer.gov/reporting/ctc.html.

[40] Wollenberg A, Moosmann N, Klein E,et al. A tool for scoring of acneiform skin eruptions induced by EGF receptor inhibition. *Exp. Dermatol.* 2008;17:790-792.

[41] Lacouture ME, Maithand ML, Saegart S, et al. A propsed EGFR inhibitor adverse event-specific grading scale from the MASCC skin toxicity study group. *Support Care Cancer* 2010;18:509-522.

[42] Cvetanovic A, Vrbic S, Filipovic S, Pejcic I, Milenkovic D, Zivkovic N, Kostic M, Petkovic I. Clinical benefit of cetuximab and prognostic value of cetuximab-related skin toxicity in metastatic colorectal cancer: a single institution analysis. *JBUON* 2014;19(1):83-90.

[43] Tol J, Koopman M, Rodenburg CJ,Cats A, Creemers GJ,Schrama JG et al. A randomised phase III study on capecitabine, oxaliplatin and bevacizumab with or without cetuximab in first-line advanced colorectal cancer, the CAIRO2 study of the Dutch Colorectal Cancer Group (DCCG). An interim analysis of toxicity. *Ann Oncol.* 2008 Apr;19(4):734-738.

[44] Sobrero AF, Maurel J, Fehrenbacher L, et al. EPIC: phase III trial of cetuximab plus irinotecan after fluoropyrimidine and oxaliplatin failure in patients with metastatic colorectal cancer. *J. Clin. Oncol* 2008;26 (14):2311–2319.

[45] Jonker DJ, O'Callaghan CJ, Karapetis CS, et al. Cetuximab for the treatment of colorectal cancer. *N. Engl. J. Med.* 2007;357(20):2040–2048.

[46] Van Cutsem E, Kohne CH, Hitre E, et al. Cetuximab and chemotherapy as initial treatment for metastatic colorectal cancer.*N. Engl. J. Med* 2009;360(14):1408–1417.

[47] Cunningham D, Humblet Y, Siena S,Khayat D, Bleiberg H,Santoro A, et al. Cetuximab Monotherapy and Cetuximab plus Irinotecan in Irinotecan-Refractory Metastatic Colorectal Cancer. *N. Engl. J. Med.* 2004;351:337-345.

[48] Bokemeyer C, Bondarenko I, Hartmann JT, Braud F, Schuch G, Zubel A, et al. Efficacy according to biomarker status of cetuximab plus FOLFOX-4 as first-line treatment for metastatic colorectal cancer: the OPUS study. *Ann. Oncol.* 2011;22(7):1535-1546.

[49] Saltz LB, Lenz HJ, Kindler HL, Hochster HS,Wadler S,Hoff PM,et al. Randomized Phase II Trial of Cetuximab, Bevacizumab, and Irinotecan Compared With Cetuximab and Bevacizumab Alone in Irinotecan-Refractory Colorectal Cancer: The BOND-2 Study. *JCO* 2007;25(29):4557-4561.

[50] Bonner JA, Harari PM, Giralt J, et al.Radiotherapy plus cetuximab for squamous-cell carcinoma of the head and neck. *N. Engl. J. Med.* 2006;354(6):567–578.

[51] Vermorken JB, Mesia R, Rivera F, et al.Platinum-based chemotherapy plus cetuximab in head and neck cancer. *N. Engl. J. Med.* 2008;359(11):1116–1127.

[52] Burtness B, Goldwasser MA, Flood W, Mattar B, Forastiere AA.Phase III randomized trial of cisplatin plus placebo compared with cisplatin plus cetuximab in metastatic/recurrent head and neck cancer: an eastern cooperative oncology group study. *J. Clin. Oncol.* 2005;23(34): 8646–8654.

[53] Lynch TJ, Patel T, Dreisbach L, et al. Cetuximab and first-line taxane/carboplatin chemotherapy in advanced non-small-cell lung cancer: results of the randomized multicenter phase III trial BMS099. *J. Clin. Oncol.* 2010;28(6): 911–917.

[54] Pirker R, Pereira JR, Szczesna A, et al. Cetuximab plus chemotherapy in patients with advanced non-small-cell lung cancer (FLEX): an open-label randomised phase III trial.*Lancet* 2009;373(9674):1525–1531.

[55] Jatoi A, Green EM, Rowland Jr. KM, Sargent DJ, Alberts SR.Clinical predictors of severe cetuximab-induced rash: observations from 933 patients enrolled in north central cancer treatment group study N0147. *Oncology* 2009;77(2):120–123.

[56] Lurje G, Nagashima F, Zhang W, et al. Polymorphisms in cyclooxygenase-2 and epidermal growth factor receptor are associated with progression-free survival independent of K-ras in metastatic colorectal cancer patients treated with single-agent cetuximab.Clin *Cancer Res.* 2008;14(23):7884–7895.

[57] Klinghammer K, Knodler M, Schmittel A, Budach V, Keilholz U, Tinhofer I. Association of epidermal growth factor receptor polymorphism, skin toxicity, and outcome in patients with squamous cell carcinoma of the head and neck receiving cetuximab-docetaxel treatment. *Clin. Cancer Res.* 2010;16 (1):304–310.

[58] Vallbohmer D, Zhang W, Gordon M, et al. Molecular determinants of cetuximab efficacy. *J. Clin. Oncol.* 2005;23(15):3536–3544.

[59] Stintzing S, Kapaun C, Laubender RP et al. Prognostic value of cetuximab-related skin toxicity in metastatic colorectal cancer patients and its correlation with parameters of the epidermal growth factor receptor signal transduction pathway: results from a randomized trial of the GERMAN AIO CRC Study Group. *Int. J. Cancer.* 2013;132:236–245.

[60] Lenz HJ, Van Cutsem E, Khambata-Ford S, et al. Multicenter phase II and translational study of cetuximab in metastatic colorectal carcinoma refractory to irinotecan, oxaliplatin, and fluoropyrimidines. *J. Clin. Oncol.* 2006; 24: 4914–4921.

[61] Boccia RV, Cosgriff TM, Headley DL, Badarinath S, and Dakhil SR. A phase II trial of FOLFOX6 and cetuximab in the first-line treatment of patients with metastatic colorectal cancer. *Clin. Colorectal Cancer.* 2010;9:102–107.

[62] Hitt R, Irigoyen A, Cortes-Funes H, Grau JJ, García-Sáenz JA, and Cruz-Hernandez JJ. Spanish Head and Neck Cancer Cooperative Group (TTCC) Phase II study of the combination of cetuximab and weekly paclitaxel in the first-line treatment of patients

with recurrent and/or metastatic squamous cell carcinoma of head and neck. *Ann. Oncol.* 2012; 23: 1016–1022.

[63] Maubec E, Petrow P, Scheer-Senyarich I, et al. Phase II study of cetuximab as first-line single-drug therapy in patients with unresectable squamous cell carcinoma of the skin. *J. Clin. Oncol.* 2011;29:3419–3426.

[64] Fleming MT, Sonpavde G, Kolodziej M, et al. Association of rash with outcomes in a randomized phase II trial evaluating cetuximab in combination with mitoxantrone plus prednisone after docetaxel for metastatic castration-resistant prostate cancer. *Clin Genitourin Cancer.* 2012;10:6–14.

[65] Burtness B, Goldwasser MA, Flood W, Mattar B, and Forastiere AA. Eastern Cooperative Oncology Group Phase III randomized trial of cisplatin plus placebo compared with cisplatin plus cetuximab in metastatic/recurrent head and neck cancer: an Eastern Cooperative Oncology Group study. *J. Clin. Oncol.* 2005;23:8646–8654.

[66] Bonner JA, Harari PM, Giralt J. et al. Radiotherapy plus cetuximab for locoregionally advanced head and neck cancer: 5-year survival data from a phase 3 randomised trial, and relation between cetuximab-induced rash and survival. *Lancet Oncol.* 2010;11:21–28.

[67] Gatzemeier U, von Pawel J, Vynnychenko I. et al. First-cycle rash and survival in patients with advanced non-small-cell lung cancer receiving cetuximab in combination with first-line chemotherapy: a subgroup analysis of data from the FLEX phase 3 study. *Lancet Oncol.* 2011;12:30–37.

[68] Li T, Perez-Soler R. Skin toxicities associated with epidermal growth factor receptor inhibitors. *Targ. Oncol.* 2009;4:107-119.

[69] 69.Lacouture ME, Cotliar J, Mitchell EP. Clinical management of EGFRI derantologic toxicities:U.S. perspective. *Oncology* 2007;21(suppl 5):17-21.

[70] Pinto C, Barone CA, Girolomoni G, Russi EG, Merlano MC,et al. Management of skin toxicity associated with cetuximab treatment in combination with chemotherapy or radiotherapy. *The Oncologist* 2011;16:228-238.

[71] Galimont-Collen AFS, Vos LE, Lavrijesn APM, Ouwerkerk J,Gelderblom H. Classification and management of skin, hair, nail and mucosal side-effects of epidermal growth factor receptor (EGFR) inhibitors. *European Journal of Cancer* 2007;43: 845-851.

[72] Fakih M, Vincent M. Adverse events associated with anti-EGFR therapies for the treatment of metastatic colorectal cancer. *Current Oncology* 2010;17(1):S18-S30.

[73] 73.Melosky B, Burkes R, Rayson D, Alcindor T, Shear N et Lacouture M. Management of skin rash during EGFR-targeted monoclonal antibody treatment for gastrointestinal malignancies:Canadian recommendation.*Current Oncology* 2009;16(1):14-24.

[74] 74. Baasa JM, Krensb LL,Guchelaarb HJ, Ouwerkerk J,De Jongc FA, Lavrijsend APM,et al. Recommendations on management of EGFR inhibitor-induced skin toxicity: A systematic review. *Cancer Treatment* Reviews 2012;38(5):505-515.

[75] 75. Scope A, Agero AL. Dusza SW, et al. Randomized double-blind trial of prophylactic oral minocycline and topical tazarotene for cetuximab-associated acne-like eruption. *J. Clin. Oncol.* 2007;25(34):5390-5396.

In: Head and Neck Cancer
Editor: Madison R. Hall
ISBN: 978-1-63482-113-1

Chapter 8

Assessment of Prognostic Factors Affecting the Treatment of Laryngeal Cancer

Alexander Karatzanis, MD, PhD *
and Maria Doulaptsi, MD
Department of Otorhinolaryngology, University of Crete School of Medicine, Heraklion, Crete, Greece

Abstract

Laryngeal cancer is the second most common type of head and neck cancer worldwide. There exist many management options for laryngeal tumors today. Besides cure, organ preservation with retaining of function has been added as a primary goal of treatment. Numerous prognostic factors regarding patients undergoing treatment for laryngeal lesions have been evaluated in the literature.

Choice of treatment may be regarded as a major factor affecting prognosis. Multiple options are available for the management of laryngeal cancer. In the treatment of advanced cases, significant changes have been noted in recent years with a clear shift toward non-surgical, organ-preservation strategies.

As there appears to be worsening survival for laryngeal cancer, it has been proposed this may be related to the shift from surgery to chemoradiation.

For cases undergoing surgical treatment the prognostic significance of surgical margins cannot be overemphasized. It is common knowledge among surgeons that the aim of any tumor surgery with therapeutic intent should be histologically confirmed disease-free margins. It has been established that patients with laryngeal cancer exhibiting compromised margins have significantly higher rates of local recurrence and even show decreased survival. Status of surgical margins significantly affects oncologic

* Corresponding author: Alexander Karatzanis, MD, PhD, Department of Otorhinolaryngology, University Hospital of Crete, 71110, Heraklion, Crete, Greece. Tel: 00306934325130, fax: 0030542106, e-mail: akaratzanis@yahoo.com.

outcome regardless of accompanying disease stage. Prognostic significance of tumor margins following laser resection shows more controversial outcomes.

Besides status of margins, N and T classification are widely considered to be significant prognostic factors. Comorbidity is an important factor affecting survival of patients with laryngeal malignancies. Age appears to be another prognostic factor although it has not proved to be independent. Same goes for the primary site of laryngeal cancer. Prognosis has traditionally been poorer for supraglottic carcinomas, compared to glottic lesions, due to the rich lymphatic drainage system and the relatively late appearance of symptoms. Histological grade of tumor has also been widely studied as a prognostic variable. Progression of dedifferentiation tends to worsen prognosis. The impact of tobacco use and alcohol consumption during treatment is still controversial. Studies have reported that long-term smoking is an independent factor of laryngeal cancer progression, and alcohol intake appears to have a well-known synergistic effect.

Lately, clinical trials have investigated the impact of viruses to prognostic outcome of laryngeal carcinomas. Accordingly, Human Papilloma virus status, specifically p16 strain, may be taken into account when considering organ preservation treatment for locally advanced larynngeal cancer. Patients with HPV/p16+ tumors have been shown to do favorably with chemoradiation, with improvement of disease specific survival (DSS) and local recurrence. Research for predictive value of biomarkers, and their impact on treatment decision making is still ongoing. Cyclin D1 expression in laryngeal cancer affects DSS and overall survival (OS).

Overexpression of EGFR is a poor prognostic factor, while low expression of BAK and NFκB were associated with good response in induction chemotherapy and chemoradiation respectively.

As many variables are considered significant in the management of laryngeal cancer, continuous evaluation may serve as a guide for more effective treatment strategies.

Introduction

Laryngeal cancer is the second most common type of head and neck cancer worldwide. According to the American Cancer Society an estimated 12.630 new cases will be diagnosed in the United States in 2014 and 3.610 patients will die from their disease [1]. Squamous cell carcinoma (SCC) is the predominant type, and approximately 40% of patients present with advanced stage disease [2]. There exist many management options for laryngeal tumors today. Besides cure, organ preservation with retaining of function has been added as a primary goal of treatment. Numerous prognostic factors regarding patients undergoing treatment for laryngeal lesions have been evaluated in the literature.

Treatment Modality

Choice of treatment may be regarded as a major factor affecting prognosis. Multiple options are available for the management of laryngeal cancer nowadays. In order to define the ideal treatment option, different aspects should be considered. These include oncologic outcomes, functional results, morbidity, as well as financial cost. Moreover, patient factors, local expertise, rehabilitation services and availability of appropriate support should be taken into consideration in treatment selection. Regarding early stage laryngeal carcinomas (Stage I, II), as defined by the American Joint Committee on Cancer 2010 (AJCC) and International

Union for Cancer Control (UICC) classification, single modality treatment is thought to be effective [3, 4]. Patients may be treated with radiation or larynx preservation surgery with similar survival outcomes. Although, there are no randomized trials in which surgery is compared to radiation with respect to local control (LC), overall survival (OS) and functional outcomes, prospective and retrospective cohort studies have shown comparable rates [5, 6]. For locally advanced laryngeal lesions (Stage III-IV) numerous management approaches have been used [7, 8]. Total laryngectomy followed by adjuvant radiation therapy has been widely considered the standard treatment option for many years [9, 10]. However, a shift toward organ preservation strategies with the use of primary chemoradiation has been recently noted [4, 9]. The American Society of Clinical Oncology (ASCO) has recommended that all patients should be evaluated regarding their suitability for a larynx-preservation approach, with total laryngectomy reserved for salvage treatment after failure of non-surgical management approaches. Among organ-preserving modalities, concurrent chemoradiotherapy demonstrated to offer significantly higher cure rates, while cisplatin is considered the chemotherapy agent of choice [4]. Nevertheless, no larynx-preservation approach has been shown to have a survival advantage compared to total laryngectomy and adjuvant radiation. In recent years there seems to appear a decreasing trend of overall survival in patients with laryngeal carcinoma [11]. It has been proposed that this may be related to the shift from surgery to chemoradiation. Additionally, recent studies have showed statistically better prognosis in terms of overall survival (OS), and disease specific survival (DSS) in patients who received surgery and adjuvant RT or CRT compared to primary CRT for advanced laryngeal cancer [8, 10, 12]. This is more evident in cases with invasion of the thyroid cartilage which are thought to be better served with initial surgery, and therefore patients with these tumors are considered poor candidates for organ sparring treatment modalities (4). Additionally, surgery seems to gain the upper hand in patients who are physically unfit to receive chemoradiation, in cases of unreliable patients and in underserved areas [9]. It must be kept in mind that primary surgery in advanced stages, specifically in T4 lesions, should not be addressed as a single modality treatment but rather be included as the initial part of combined strategy followed always by radiotherapy and in many cases by chemotherapy as well.

Surgical Margins

Surgical treatment of laryngeal cancer includes external total or partial surgery and more recently transolar laser surgery [13]. Whenever surgical management is selected and no matter which type is used, the significance of achieving tumor-free surgical margins cannot be overstressed [14]. It has been established that patients with head and neck cancer exhibiting positive resection margins have significantly higher rates of local and regional recurrence and even show decreased survival. With regard to laryngeal cancer LC, DSS and OS have been found to be statistically superior for patients with negative surgical margins (Ro) compared to patients with compromised borders (R+) in numerous studies [14-20]. Impact of margin status on survival remains significant even when cases with early (Stage I, II) and advanced (Stage III, IV) stage of disease are separately evaluated. Consequently, status of surgical margins significantly affects oncologic outcomes regardless of accompanying disease stage [12, 14, 18, 20]. Positive histologic borders left untreated have distinct prognostic relevance in squamous cell carcinoma of the larynx and have been found to be more often associated with advanced T classification carcinomas. Moreover, status of surgical margins constantly emerges as an independent prognostic factor in multivariate analyses on clinical trials. Therefore, the aim of any tumor surgery with therapeutic intent should be histologically confirmed disease-free borders. However, definition of an oncologically safe resection remains an issue under debate and seems to depend on the anatomic site. Specifically, wide surgical margins seem to be of minor importance in laryngeal cancer as these have not been associated with better local control rates [8, 21]. In addition, wide margins have a negative effect on functional outcome when organ preservation surgery is performed.

Regarding early laryngeal cancer several laryngeal-preserving techniques are available. Such techniques aim to cure patients while obtaining optimal functional outcome and include transoral laser CO2 microsurgery (TLM) as well as open procedures. Laryngofissure with cordectomy, vertical partial laryngectomy, and frontolateral partial laryngectomy were in use extensively in the past but have been largely replaced by endoscopic laser surgery [22]. Transoral laser CO2 microsurgery represents a minimally invasive surgical approach which allows tumors to be removed with minimal sacrifice of healthy tissue and with retention of acceptable quality of voice [17].

Transcervical approaches have shown comparable treatment outcomes, in terms of LC and DSS with laser surgery. However, TLM appears to have low morbidity and mortality, shorter periods of hospitalization, lower cost, and its functional results are generally considered superior to those of open surgery [22]. Moreover, the use of TLM in laryngeal cancer treatment offers significant advantages with regard to margin control, as it allows easy, repeated and direct access to the tumor site [14, 23, 24]. This technique is therefore, ideal for additional sessions whenever surgical margins are found compromised. With the application of TLM the impact of negative margins on prognosis does not seem to be affected by the number of procedures necessary in order to achieve such margins since it is not the number but the final histologic status that actually affects prognosis [15, 16, 21].

Therefore, incomplete tumor resection may easily be managed with revision surgery [15, 16, 18].

With regard to TLM specifically, however, prognostic significance of tumor borders shows more controversial outcomes. Laser surgery may cause increased difficulties in order for pathologists to access the status of surgical margins [13, 17, 23].

These are related to the nature of laser CO2 itself and include tissue contraction, evaporation, carbonization, heat artifacts, small sample size and orientation. Such difficulties often result in surgical margins falsely assessed as positive or undetermined on permanent histology. However, favorable prognostic outcomes have been reported even in cases where surgical borders had not been clearly justified on permanent histology. Specifically, compromised and uncertain margins were not related with recurrence or poor oncologic outcomes, whenever second look procedure or close follow up were selected [25-27]. Frozen section control is used in order to supplant difficulties in assessing status of surgical margins. However, as many institutions worldwide do not routinely rely on frozen section for practical reasons, a philosophy of selective second look procedure or a "watch and wait" strategy have been favored in cases of discrepancy between surgeon's clinical impression and histopathology regarding the completeness of resection. For T1 glottic lesions undergoing

TLM with curative intent, it has been recently proposed that whenever the surgeon is confident that the resection borders are satisfactory and no further treatment is required, cases may be managed with close follow up, even if positive or suspicious margins are mentioned in the pathology report [25-27].

TNM Staging

TNM is a cancer staging notation system introduced by UICC and AJCC, in order to categorize and classify universally patients with malignant lesions based on the size and extension of a primary lesion (T), its regional lymphatic drainage (N), and distant metastases (M) [3, 4]. The prognostic significance of TNM staging is high and may not be overlooked. Different therapeutic approaches have been developed for different stages. Survival of patients with laryngeal cancer drops as the stage increases.

Specifically, the survival rate of early laryngeal cancer (Stages I, II) is estimated at 73% to 92% while for advanced stages (III, IV) only 35% to 64% [28]. Primary tumor size and extension (T) significantly affects prognosis to the majority of prospective and retrospective large series studies [7-12, 17, 18]. Moreover, T staging is used as guide for selection of the proper therapeutic strategy. Invasion of thyroid cartilage and large tumor volumetry exceeding 15cm have been related with poor response in patients who received definitive CRT [4, 29]. They have also been associated with lower locoregional control (LCR), DSS and OS.

Therefore, these patients are considered poor candidates for a larynx preservation approach [4]. Primary surgery, usually total laryngectomy is recommended in this setting. Interestingly, there are studies suggesting that tumor volumetry may be more important than T stage in prediction of DSS and OS in laryngeal squamous cell carcinoma [29].

Status of regional lymph nodes is, along with surgical margins, the factor which constantly declares independence in multivariate analyses on clinical trials. In fact, it has been suggested that cervical lymph node metastasis is the most important prognostic factor, as studies have shown a decrease of about 50% in OS with its presence [12, 18, 19, 28, 30]. However, clinical stage combines the effects of both tumor extend and lymph node metastasis on prognosis. Statistical significance of N classification emphasizes the need for timely diagnosis and management especially of glottic cancer, since regional disease is quite uncommon during the early stages.

Primary Site

The impact of primary site in laryngeal cancer prognosis has been established in univariate analyses; however, it is not considered an independent prognostic factor. Prognosis has traditionally been poorer for supraglottic carcinomas due to the rich lymphatic drainage system and the relatively late appearance of symptoms. Moreover, supraglottic carcinomas are prone to occult lymph node metastasis. These factors make early diagnosis difficult and lead to poorer prognosis [31]. In contrast, due to the sparse lymphatics of the glottis and early symptom of persistent hoarseness associated with glottic carcinoma, most cases may be diagnosed at an early stage, and therefore, have better prognosis [8, 21]. With regard to glottic malignancies the impact of anterior commissure involvement in prognosis remains controversial. Nevertheless, most authors agree that anterior commissure involvement pertains a worse prognosis [32-34].

Tumor Histology

Tumor grade is an indicator of how quickly tumor cells may spread. Generally, there are four grades in cancer histology, covering a wide spectrum from 'well differentiated' (low grade) tumor cells with a slow pattern of growth, to 'undifferentiated' (high grade) where tumors tend to grow faster and spread more rapidly than low grade tumors. Histological grade of tumor has also been widely studied as a prognostic variable. Progression of dedifferentiation tends to worsen prognosis [3]. However, tumor histology has not been shown to constitute an independent prognostic factor.

Tobacco and Alcohol

Avoidance of tobacco and alcohol consumption in general may prevent 90% of laryngeal malignancies. The impact of tobacco use and alcohol consumption on laryngeal cancer prognosis, however, is still controversial. Studies in several populations have reported that long-term smoking is an independent factor of laryngeal cancer progression, with direct dose-related effect on SCC, as well as a benefit of cessation. Prospective, non-randomized, and retrospective trials have shown that continuation of smoking significantly affects overall survival rate [2, 35, 36]. Alcohol consumption seems to have a multiplicative effect on laryngeal cancer and relative risk is higher for supraglottis rather than glottis. In contrast, the impact of increased relative risk for tobacco use is higher for glottic than supraglottic SCC.

However, several studies have failed to statistically correlate tobacco and alcohol intake with laryngeal cancer prognosis [18, 19]. Nevertheless, smoking during radiation treatment has proven to be a negative predictive factor. Therefore, patients should be encouraged to quit smoking immediately after diagnosis and throughout treatment [4].

Biomarkers

Low cure rates and morbidity following surgical treatment for advanced laryngeal cancer, as well as failure of chemoradiation to improve overall survival generated the need to identify molecular pathways involved in treatment response and resistance. Biomarkers have received increasing attention, for their role not only in carcinogenesis but also as predictive factors for treatment decision, recurrence and survival. A large panel of molecular markers have been studied in clinical trials. Among these, p53, EGFR, VEGF, cyclin D1, BAK, Bcl-2, Bcl- xl, NFκB, CD24, Ki-67 are the most important. With regard to overall outcome, cyclin D1 and CD24 may be considered as statistically significant prognostic factors. Specifically, cyclin D1 expression is associated with low overall survival rate while CD24 with lower risk of death

[37]. Regarding disease specific survival (DSS), cyclin D1 and EGFR (Epidermal Growth Factor Receptor) are related with poor rates. Biomarkers have been used in clinical trials in order to identify patients who do not respond in chemoradiation and will be best treated surgically. Notably, overexpression of BAK, Bcl-2, Bcl-xl, and cytoplasmic NFκB have been associated with poor response to laryngeal preservation modality treatment [37, 38]. The p53 is a tumor suppressor protein showing some kind of mutation in approximately 50% of head and neck cancers. Moreover, it has been suggested that expression of positive p53 phenotype may predict lower OS and locoregional control [38, 39]. However, larger, prospective clinical trials are necessary in order to integrate these markers as part of molecular staging, and as predictors for organ preservation and other oncological outcomes.

Viruses

Recent emerging data have demonstrated a relationship between HNSCC and Human Papilloma (HPV) genotypes. It has been indicated that HPV related HNSCC defines a unique entity with distinct biology, which should be treated separately, is more responsive to chemoradiation and shows improved survival, with 60% lower risk of death. This has been primarily established for oropharyngeal cancer [40].

Lately, however, clinical trials have attempted to investigate the impact of these viruses on the prognostic outcome of laryngeal carcinomas. The most common type of HPV detected in laryngeal carcinoma is p16 strain, while p18 is the second most common. In contrast to squamous cell carcinoma of the oropharynx, many studies have failed to detect a clear association between HPV status and clinical outcome of laryngeal cancer [41-43].

Recently, however, in a case series study of patients with advanced laryngeal carcinoma, HPV/p16+ tumors were managed more favorably with chemoradiation compared to surgical treatment, with improvement of DSS and locoregional control [44]. It has been suggested, therefore, that HPV/p16 status may be taken into account when considering organ preservation in locally advanced laryngeal cancer.

Nevertheless, further studies are needed in order to clarify the impact of viruses in prognostic outcome in laryngeal carcinomas.

Age, Sex

Whether age affects oncologic outcomes in laryngeal cancer is still under debate. Many studies demonstrated age as significant prognostic factor for survival in univariate analyses [18, 19]. However, age constantly fails to emerge as an independent prognostic factor in multivariate analyses. Nevertheless, a multicentre cohort study in Germany showed that age at first diagnosis was the most important predictive factor for overall survival in multivariate analysis [45, 46]. In general, although patients of older age experience worse survival rates than younger subjects, deviation is not statistically significant. Regarding the impact of sex in survival, clinical trials have failed to demonstrate statistically significant improvement in oncological outcomes for female or male subjects. Disease specific survival was only found to be better in female patients who received no surgical treatment for advanced (stage III) laryngeal SCC [10].

Comorbidity

The presence of additional illness unrelated to the tumor has been found to play a role in head and neck cancer outcome. Moreover, comorbidity in laryngeal carcinomas has been shown to negatively influence overall survival [47, 48]. Patients with additional health problems were more likely to receive surgical treatment than chemoradiationfor laryngeal cancer. Different tools have been used to quantify comorbidity. Adult Comorbidity Evaluation 27 (ACE27), Charlson Comorbidity Index (CCI), Karnofsky Performance Status Scale (KPSS), and Cumulative Illness Rating Scale have been the most frequently used. Karnofsky status ≤ 80 has been independently associated with OS and DSS. Similarly, ACE $27 \geq 2$ has been found to have a negative impact on overall survival [49]. Among these instruments, ACE 27 is a more reliable predictor of survival in laryngeal cancer [50].

References

[1] *American Cancer Society: Cancer Facts and Figures 2014*. Atlanta, Ga: American Cancer Society, 2014.

[2] Chu, E. A. 1., Kim, Y. J. Laryngeal cancer: diagnosis and preoperative work-up. *Otolaryngol. Clin. Nor. Am.* 2008 Aug.;41(4):673-95,v.doi: 10. 1016/j.otc.2008.01.016.

[3] American Joint Committee on Cancer (AJCC). *Manual for staging of cancer.* 7th edition. New York, NY; Springer-Verlag; 2010:30-38.

[4] American Society of Clinical Oncology1, Pfister, D. G., Laurie, S. A., Weinstein, G. S., Mendenhall, W. M., Adelstein, D. J., Ang, K. K., Clayman, G. L., Fisher, S. G., Forastiere, A. A., Harrison, L. B., Lefebvre, J. L., Leupold, N., List, M. A., O'Malley, B. O., Patel, S., Posner, M. R., Schwartz, M. A., Wolf, G. T. American Society of Clinical Oncology clinical practice guideline for the use of larynx-preservation strategies in the treatment of laryngeal cancer. *J. Clin. Oncol.* 2006 Aug. 1;24(22):3693-704.

[5] Higgins, K. M., Shah, M. D., Ogaick, M. J., Enepekides, D. Treatment of early-stage glottic cancer: meta-analysis comparison of laser excision versus radiotherapy. *Journal of Otolaryngology - Head and Neck Surgery* 2009; 38(6): 603-612.

[6] Higgins, K. M. What treatment for early-stage glottic carcinoma among adult patients: CO2 endolaryngeal laser excision versus standard fractionated external beam radiation is superior in terms of cost utility? *Laryngoscope.* 2011 Jan.;121(1):116-34. doi: 10.1002/lary.21226.

[7] Sessions, D. G., Lenox, J., Spector, G. J., Newland, D., Simpson, J., Haughey, B. H., Chao, K. S. Management of T3N0M0 glottic carcinoma: therapeutic outcomes. *Laryngose.* 2002 Jul.;112(7 Pt 1): 1281-8.

[8] Spector, G. J., Sessions, D. G., Lenox, J., Newland, D., Simpson, J., Haughey, B. H. Management of stage IV glottic carcinoma: therapeutic outcomes. *Laryngoscope*. 2004 Aug.;114(8):1438-46.

[9] Silver, C. E. 1., Beitler, J. J., Shaha, A. R., Rinaldo, A., Ferlito, A. Current trends in initial management of laryngeal cancer: the declining use of open surgery. *Eur. Arch. Otorhinolaryngol.* 2009 Sep.;266(9): 1333-52. doi: 10.1007/s00405-009-1028-2. Epub. 2009 Jul. 14.

[10] Megwalu, U. C., Sikora, A. G. Survival outcomes in advanced laryngeal cancer. *JAMA Otolaryng. Head Neck Surg.* 2014 Sep.;140(9):85560.doi: 10.1001/jamaoto.2014.1671.

[11] Hoffman, H. T. 1., Porter, K., Karnell, L. H., Cooper, J. S., Weber, R. S., Langer, C. J., Ang, K. K., Gay, G., Stewart, A., Robinson, R. A. Laryngeal cancer in the United States: changes in demographics, patterns of care, and survival. *Laryngoscope*. 2006 Sep.;116(9 Pt 2 Suppl. 111):1-13.

[12] Karatzanis, A. D., Psychogios, G., Waldfahrer, F., Kapsreiter, M., Zenk, J., Velegrakis, G. A., Iro, H. Management of locally advanced laryngeal cancer. *J. Otolaryngol. Head Neck Surg*. 2014 Jan. 28;43:4. doi: 10. 1186/1916-0216-43-4.

[13] Batsakis, J. G. Surgical margins in squamous cell carcinomas. *Ann. Otol. Rhinol. Laryngol.* 1988;124:1245-214.

[14] Tufano, R. P. 1., Stafford, E. M. Organ preservation surgery for laryngeal cancer. *Otolaryngol. Clin. North Am*. 2008 Aug.;41(4):741-55, vi. doi: 10.1016/j.otc .2008.01.020.

[15] Jäckel, M. C. 1., Ambrosch, P., Martin, A., Steiner, W. Impact of re-resection for inadequate margins onthe prognosis of upper aerodigestive tract cancer treated by laser microsurgery. *Laryngoscope*. 2007 Feb.; 117 (2):350-6.

[16] Karatzanis, A. D. 1., Waldfahrer, F., Psychogios, G., Hornung, J., Zenk, J., Velegrakis, G. A., Iro, H. Effect of repeated laser microsurgical operations on laryngeal cancer prognosis. *Head Neck*. 2010 Jul.;32(7): 921-8. doi: 10.1002/hed.21272.

[17] Iro, H., Waldfahrer, F., Altendorf-Hofmann, A., Weidenbecher, M., Sauer, R., Steiner, W. Transoral laser surgery of supraglottic cancer: follow-up of 141 patients. *Arch. Otolaryngol. Head Neck Surg*. 1998 Nov.;124(11):1245-50.

[18] Karatzanis, A. D. 1., Waldfahrer, F., Psychogios, G., Hornung, J., Zenk, J., Velegrakis, G. A., Iro, H. Resection margins and other prognostic factors regarding surgically treated glottic carcinomas. Resection margins and other prognostic factors regarding surgically treated glottic carcinomas.

[19] Zhang, S. Y., Lu, Z. M., Luo, X. N., Chen, L. S., Ge, P. J., Song, X. H., Chen, S. H., Wu, Y. L. Retrospective analysis of prognostic factors in 205 patients with laryngeal squamous cell carcinoma who underwent surgical treatment. *PLoS One*. 2013 Apr. 4;8(4):e60157. doi: 10.1371/ journal.pone.0060157.

[20] Zhao, H. 1., Ren, J., Zhuo, X., Ye, H., Zou, J., Liu, S. Prognostic significance of Survivin and CD44v6 in laryngeal cancer surgical margins. *J. Cancer Res. Clin. Oncol.* 2008 Oct.;134(10):1051-8. doi: 10.1007/s00432-008-0391-5.

[21] Roh, J. L. 1., Kim, D. H., Park, C. I. The utility of second-look operation after laser microresection of glottic carcinoma involving the anterior commissure. *Laryngoscope.* 2008 Aug.;118(8):1400-4. doi: 10.1097/ MLG.0b013e318175338f.

[22] Karatzanis, A. D., Psychogios, G., Zenk, J., Waldfahrer, F., Hornung, J., Velegrakis, G. A., Iro, H. Comparison among different available surgical approaches in T1 glottic cancer. *Laryngoscope*. 2009 Sep.;119(9):1704-8. doi: 10.1002/lary.20537.

[23] Absolon, K. B., Keshishian, J. First laryngectomy for cancer as performed by Theodor Billroth on December 31, 1873: a hundred anniversary. *Rev. Surg.* 1974 Mar.-Apr.;31(2):65-70.

[24] Steiner, W. Experience in endoscopic surgery of malignant tumors of the upper aerodigestive tract. *Adv. Otorhinolaryngol.* 1988;39:135-144.

[25] Michel, J., Fakhry, N., Duflo, S., Lagier, A., Mancini, J., Dessi, P., Giovanni, A. Prognostic value of the status of resection margins after endoscopic laser cordectomy for T1a glottic carcinoma. *Eur. Ann. Otorhinolaryngol. Head Neck Dis*. 2011;128(6): 297-300. doi:10.1016/j. anorl.2011.05.006.

[26] Hartl, D. M., de Monès, E., Hans, S., Janot, F., Brasnu, D. Treatment of early stage glottic cancer by transoral laser resection. *Ann. Otol. Rhinol. Laryngol.* 2007;116(11):832-6.

[27] Peretti, G., Nicolai, P., De Zinis, L. O. R., et al. Endoscopic CO2 laser excision for Tis, T1, and T2 glottic carcinomas: cure rate and prognostic factors. *Otolaryngol. Head Neck Surg*. 2000;123: 124-31. Brondbo, K., Fridrich, K., Boysen, M. Laser surgery of T1a glottic carcinomas; significance of resection margins. *Eur. Arch. Otorhinolaryngol.* 2007; 264:627-630.

[28] Jose, J. 1., Coatesworth, A. P., Johnston, C., MacLennan, K. Cervical node metastases in squamous cell carcinoma of the upper aerodigestive tract: the significance of extracapsular spread and soft tissue deposits. *Head Neck*. 2003 Jun.;25(6):451-6.

[29] Hsin, L. J. 1., Fang, T. J., Tsang, N. M., Chin, S. C., Yen, T. C., Li, H. Y., Liao, C. T., Chen, I. H. Tumor volumetry as a prognostic factor in the management of T4a laryngeal cancer. *Laryngoscope*. 2014 May; 124 (5):1134-40. doi: 10.1002/lary.24461. Epub. 2013 Nov. 19.

[30] Markou, K. 1., Goudakos, J., Triaridis, S., Konstantinidis, J., Vital, V., Nikolaou, A. The role of tumor size and patient's age as prognostic factors in laryngeal cancer. *Hippokratia*. 2011 Jan.;15(1):75-80.

[31] Liu, T. R. 1., Yang, A. K., Chen, F. J., Zeng, M. S., Song, M., Guo, Z. M., Chen, W. K., Ouyang, D., Li, Q. L., Chen, Y. F., Zhang, Q., Zeng, Z. Y. [Survival and prognostic analysis of 221 patients with advanced laryngeal squamous cell carcinoma treated by surgery]. *Ai Zheng*. 2009 Mar.;28(3):297-302.

[32] Steiner, W. 1., Ambrosch, P., Rödel, R. M., Kron, M. Impact of anterior commissure involvement on local control of early glottic carcinoma treated by laser microresection. *Laryngoscope*. 2004 Aug.;114(8):1485-91.

[33] Eckel, H. E. Local recurrences following transoral laser surgery for early glottic carcinoma: frequency, management, and outcome. *Ann. Otol. Rhinol. Laryngol.* 2001 Jan.;110(1):7-15.

[34] Kasapoğlu, F. 1., Erişen, L., Erdoğan, C. Suspicion of cricohyoidopexy line rupture after supracricoid partial laryngectomy and the value of computed tomography to exclude this complication. *Kulak Burun Bogaz Ihtis Derg.* 2008 May-Jun.;18(3):179-81.

[35] Kikidis, D. 1., Vlastarakos, P. V., Manolopoulos, L., Yiotakis, I. Continuation of smoking after treatment of laryngeal cancer: an independent prognostic factor?. *ORL J.*

Otorhinolaryngol. Relat. Spec. 2012;74(5):250-4. doi: 10.1159/000342685. Epub. 2012 Oct. 13.

[36] Boffetta, P. 1., Merletti, F., Faggiano, F., Migliaretti, G., Ferro, G., Zanetti, R., Terracini, B. Prognostic factors and survival of laryngeal cancer patients from Turin, Italy. A population-based study. *Am. J. Epidemiol.* 1997 Jun. 15;145(12):1100-5.

[37] Bradford, C. R. 1., Kumar, B., Bellile, E., Lee, J., Taylor, J., D'Silva, N., Cordell, K., Kleer, C., Kupfer, R., Kumar, P., Urba, S., Worden, F., Eisbruch, A., Wolf, G. T., Teknos, T. N., Prince, M. E., Chepeha, D. B., Hogikyan, N. D., Moyer, J. S., Carey, T. E. Biomarkers in advanced larynx cancer. *Laryngoscope.* 2014 Jan.;124(1):179-87. doi: 10.1002/ lary.24245. Epub. 2013 Jul. 12.

[38] Małecki, K. 1., Gliński, B. 1., Mucha-Małecka, A. 1., Ryś, J. 2., Kruczak, A. 2., Roszkowski, K. 3., Urbańska-Gąsiorowska, M. 4., Hetnał, M. 1. Prognostic and predictive significance of p53, EGFr, Ki-67 in larynx preservation treatment. *Rep. Pract. Oncol. Radiother.* 2010 Aug. 3;15(4):87-92. doi: 10.1016/j.rpor.2010.06.001.

[39] Osman, I. 1., Sherman, E., Singh, B., Venkatraman, E., Zelefsky, M., Bosl, G., Scher, H., Shah, J., Shaha, A., Kraus, D., Cordon-Cardo, C., Pfister, D. G. Alteration of p53 pathway in squamous cell carcinoma of the head and neck: impact on treatment outcome in patients treated with larynx preservation intent. *J. Clin. Oncol.* 2002 Jul. 1;20(13):2980-7.

[40] Dayyani, F. 1., Etzel, C. J., Liu, M., Ho, C. H., Lippman, S. M., Tsao, A. S. Meta-analysis of the impact of human papillomavirus (HPV) on cancer risk and overall survival in head and neck squamous cell carcinomas (HNSCC). *Head Neck Oncol.* 2010 Jun. 29;2:15. doi: 10. 1186/1758-3284-2-15.

[41] Isayeva, T. 1., Li, Y., Maswahu, D., Brandwein-Gensler, M. Human papillomavirus in non-oropharyngeal head and neck cancers: a systematic literature review. *Head Neck Pathol.* 2012 Jul.;6 Suppl. 1:S104-20. doi: 10.1007/s12105-012-0368-1. Epub. 2012 Jul. 3.

[42] Ankola, A. A. 1., Smith, R. V., Burk, R. D., Prystowsky, M. B., Sarta, C., Schlecht, N. F. Comorbidity, human papillomavirus infection and head and neck cancer survival in an ethnically diverse population. *Oral Oncol.* 2013 Sep.;49(9):911-7. doi: 10.1016/j.oraloncology.2013.07.001.

[43] Chernock, R. D. 1., Wang, X., Gao, G., Lewis, J. S. Jr, Zhang, Q., Thorstad, W. L., El-Mofty, S. K. Detection and significance of human papillomavirus, CDKN2A(p16) and CDKN1A(p21) expression in squamous cell carcinoma of the larynx. *Mod. Pathol.* 2013 Feb.; 26(2): 223-31. doi: 10.1038/modpathol.2012.159.

[44] Shaughnessy, J. N. 1., Farghaly, H., Wilson, L., Redman, R., Potts, K., Bumpous, J., Silverman, C., Dunlap, N. E. HPV: a factor in organ preservation for locally advanced larynx and hypopharynx cancer? *Am. J. Otolaryngol.* 2014 Jan.-Feb.;35(1):19-24. doi: 10.1016/j.amjoto.2013. 08.006.

[45] Ramroth, H. 1., Schoeps, A., Rudolph, E., Dyckhoff, G., Plinkert, P., Lippert, B., Feist, K., Delank, K. W., Scheuermann, K., Baier, G., Ott, I., Chenouda, S., Becher, H., Dietz, A. Factors predicting survival after diagnosis of laryngeal cancer. *Oral Oncol.* 2011 Dec.;47(12):1154-8. doi: 10.1016/j.oraloncology.2011.08.003.

[46] Yilmaz, T. 1., Hoşal, S., Gedikoglu, G., Turan, E., Ayas, K. Prognostic significance of depth of invasion in cancer of the larynx. *Laryngoscope.* 1998 May;108(5):764-8.

[47] Paleri, V. 1., Wight, R. G., Silver, C. E., Haigentz, M. Jr, Takes, R. P., Bradley, P. J., Rinaldo, A., Sanabria, A., Bień, S., Ferlito, A. Comorbidity in head and neck cancer: a critical appraisal and recommendations for practice. *Oral Oncol.* 2010 Oct.;46(10):712-9. doi: 10.1016/j.oraloncology.2010.07.008.

[48] Habbous, S. 1., Harland, L. T., La Delfa, A., Fadhel, E., Xu, W., Liu, F. F., Goldstein, D., Waldron, J., Huang, S. H., O'Sullivan, B., Liu, G., Habbous, S. 1., Harland, L. T., La Delfa, A., Fadhel, E., Xu, W., Liu, F. F., Goldstein, D., Waldron, J., Huang, S. H., O'Sullivan, B., Liu, G. *Head Neck.* 2014 Jun.;36(6):802-10. doi: 10.1002/hed.23360.

[49] Sanabria, A. 1., Carvalho, A. L., Vartanian, J. G., Magrin, J., Ikeda, M. K., Kowalski, L. P. Comorbidity is a prognostic factor in elderly patients with head and neck cancer. *Ann. Surg. Oncol.* 2007 Apr.;14(4):1449-57.

[50] Nesic, V. S. 1., Petrovic, Z. M., Sipetic, S. B., Jesic, S. D., Soldatovic, I. A., Kastratovic, D. A. Comparison of the Adult Comorbidity Evaluation 27 and the Charlson Comorbidity indices in patients with laryngeal squamous cell carcinoma. *J. Laryngol. Otol.* 2012 May;126(5):516-24. doi: 10.1017/S0022215112000254.

Index

B

C

D

E

F

G

H

I

J

K

L

N

O

P

Q

R

S

U

V

W

X

Y